THE
SKIN, HAIR
& NAILS

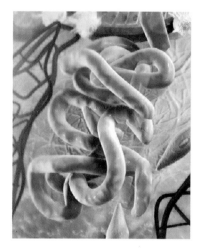

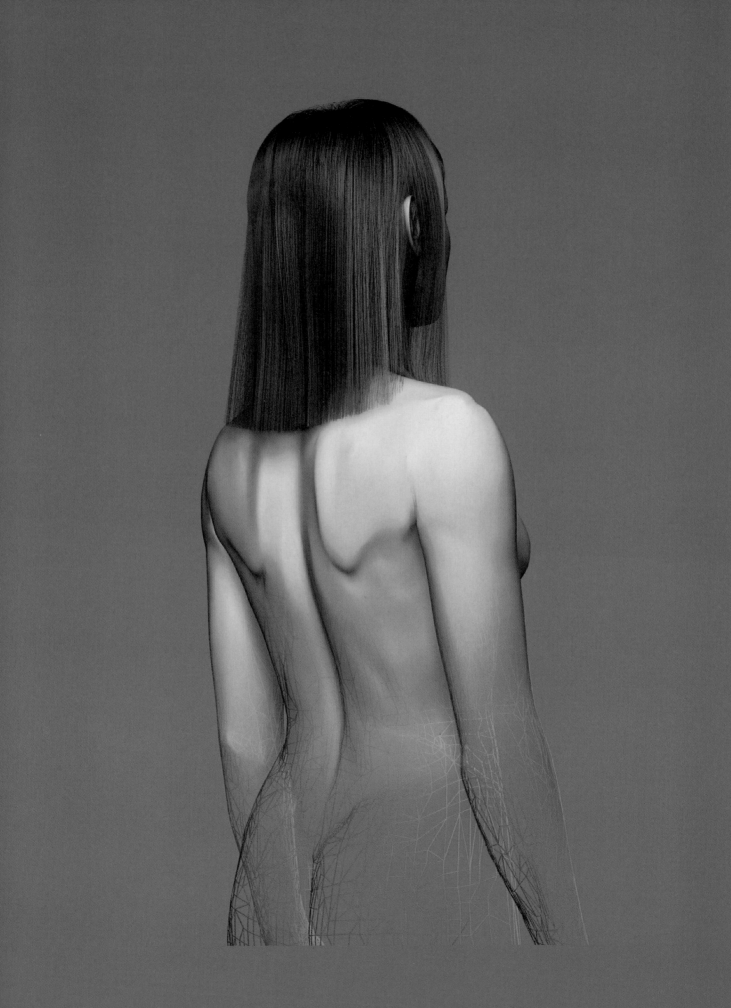

THE
SKIN, HAIR
& NAILS

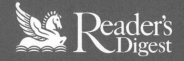

The Reader's Digest Association Limited
London New York Sydney Montreal

The Skin, Hair and Nails

was created and produced by
Carroll & Brown Limited
20 Lonsdale Road
London NW6 6RD
for Reader's Digest, London

ISBN 0 276 42704 1

Reproduced by Colour Systems, London
Printed and bound in the EEC by Arvato
Iberia.

The information in this book is for reference only; it is not intended as a substitute for a doctor's diagnosis and care. The editors urge anyone with continuing medical problems or symptoms to consult a doctor.

Managing editor
Anne Yelland

Managing art editor
Anne Fisher

Editors
Judy Fovargue, Marianne Canty, Anna Southgate

Art editors
Maxine Lea, Vimit Punater

Design assistant
Jim Cheatle

Series medical consultant
Dr Lesley Hickin, MB BS, BSc, DRCOG, MRCGP, General Practitioner

Dermatology specialist consultant
Dr Tony Chu, FRCP, Senior Lecturer, Honorary Consultant Dermatologist, Imperial College School of Medicine, Hammersmith Campus, London

CONTRIBUTORS

Wynnie Chan, BSc, PhD, Public Health Nutritionist

Dr Sandeep H Cliff, MB, BSc, MRCP, Consultant Dermatologist, Honorary Senior Lecturer, Surrey

Mr Brian Coghlan, MD, FRCS (Plast), Consultant Plastic Surgeon, Guy's Hospital, London

F J Cunningham, MRIPH MIT (Lond), Member of the Institute of Trichologists, The Trichology Centre, Rochdale

Christel Edwards-de Graauw, Nail Technician, Nail Artist and Makeup Artist, Fingernails Direct, Northern Ireland

Dr Colin Fleming, BSc, MB ChB, MRCP, Consultant Dermatologist, Department of Dermatology, Ninewells Hospital, Dundee, Honorary Senior Lecturer, University of Dundee

Katy Glynne, BSc, MRPharmS, Dip Pharmacy Practice, Clinical Services Manager, Charing Cross Hospital, London, Clinical Lecturer, The School of Pharmacy, University of London

Dr Lesley Hickin, MB BS, BSc, DRCOG, MRCGP, General Practitioner

Dr Shona Ogilvie, MB ChB, MRCGP, Clinical Fellow, University Department of Dermatology, Ninewells Hospital, Dundee

Penny Preston, MB ChB, MRGCP, Medical Writer

Beverly Westwood, RN, BSc, MSc, Research Director to Mr Brian Coghlan

For Reader's Digest
Series Editor Christine Noble
Art Editor Julie Bennett
Reader's Digest General Books
Editorial Director Cortina Butler
Art Director Nick Clark

The Skin, Hair and Nails

Awareness of health issues and expectations of medicine are greater today than ever before. A long and healthy life has come to be looked on as not so much a matter of luck but as almost a right. However, as our knowledge of health and the causes of disease has grown, it has become increasingly clear that health is something that we can all influence, for better or worse, through choices we make in our lives. *Your Body Your Health* is designed to help you make the right choices to make the most of your health potential. Each volume in the series focuses on a different physiological system of the body, explaining what it does and how it works. There is a wealth of advice and health tips on diet, exercise and lifestyle factors, as well as the health checks you can expect throughout life. You will find out what can go wrong and what can be done about it, and learn from people's real-life experiences of diagnosis and treatment. Finally, there is a detailed A to Z index of the major conditions which can affect the system. The series builds into a complete user's manual for the care and maintenance of the entire body.

This volume examines the body's largest organ, demonstrating how the skin keeps out the hostile world and protects our internal organs. Follow the fascinating life story of skin and hair cells, and how they respond to our bodies' ageing processes. Find out how a single cell detects a featherlight touch, how the skin and hair get their colour, and why we need nails. By monitoring what is normal for your skin and hair you can gain an understanding of what threatens them, and use our guides to devise basic care regimes for the skin, hair and nails to make sure yours always look their best. Discover how important diet is for the health of skin, hair and nails, and how to ensure you get all the nutrients they need. The sun is one of the biggest threats your skin must face, so here are sensible guidelines on safety in the sun. Finally, you can read what can go wrong with the skin, who are the professionals involved in diagnosing and treating skin problems, and how drugs, light and revolutionary surgical techniques can help to put them right.

Contents

1

How your skin, hair and nails work

2

Keeping your skin, hair and nails healthy

3

What happens when things go wrong

The life story of the skin

Despite the almost universal human preoccupation with appearance, most of us do not realise that our bodies have ingenious and sophisticated features that really are just skin deep. Evolution has given us a highly specialised organ – the skin – that puts us in touch with the outside world while protecting the delicate organs inside the body from many potential dangers in our environment.

The skin is the largest organ in the body and it fulfils many vital functions. It forms a protective barrier between the body and the environment, and is an important part of the immune system, detecting infections. It helps to regulate the body's temperature, stopping us from overheating (by sweating), and it protects us from damage by ultraviolet (UV) radiation. As a sensory organ, the skin helps us to discern conditions in the outside world – temperature, texture, vibrations – and is a medium for social and sexual communication.

A failure in any one these functions can have serious consequences. If temperature regulation fails we can develop heat stroke or hypothermia. If the barrier function is affected we can lose fluid and become dehydrated. Sensory incapacity can result in physical injury, from burns to bruises, while a failure of the immune response can lead to overwhelming infection. Furthermore, because of the importance of the skin to our appearance and self-esteem, skin problems often have a social and psychological impact in addition to their medical consequences. In fact, many people with a skin problem that is not seriously harmful physically still find their lives blighted by real or perceived rejection by society.

HOW SKIN EVOLVED

Millions of years of evolutionary development were needed to produce the nude human beings we are today, with skin, hair and nails that seemingly function primarily as aids to beauty and sexual attraction. The skin is

On average, each square centimetre of skin contains 10 hairs, 15 sebaceous glands, 100 sweat glands and a metre of tiny blood vessels.

8

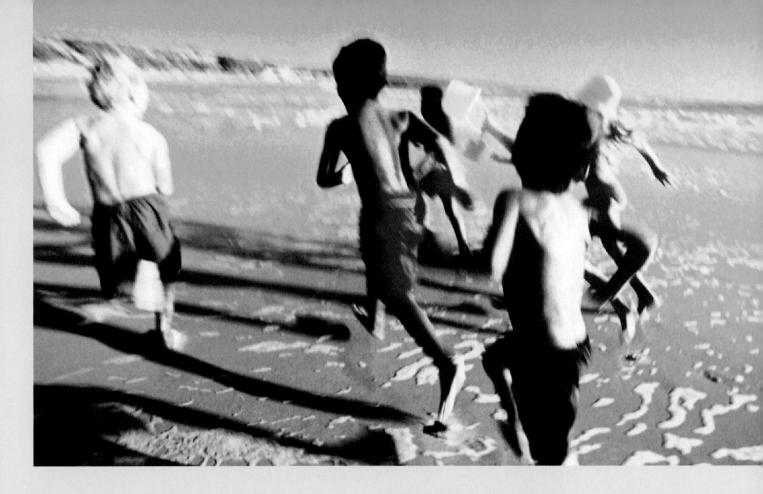

comprised of tightly packed cells arranged in two layers: the epidermis (top layer) and the dermis (lower layer). Melanocytes – specialised cells in the epidermis – give skin (and hair) its colour, but the principal role of these cells is to protect the delicate DNA in the cell nucleus from damage by ultraviolet radiation. This evolutionary step was essential once humans started to become less hairy.

WHY WE NEED HAIR

In most mammals, hair or fur plays an essential role in survival, particularly in heat conservation. This is not the case in humans. Scalp hair does function as a protection against cold, minor injury and the cancer-inducing effects of UV radiation, but its main role in human society is as an organ of display to attract a mate – hence its importance to the cosmetics industry.

HOW THE SKIN DEVELOPS

The skin, hair and nails develop early in the life of the embryo: the basal layer of the epidermis begins to develop just four weeks after conception. By seven weeks, flat cells overlying the basal layer form the periderm, which is cast

Different skin colours and hues
Skin colour is due to the amount of the pigment melanin that is in your skin. People with darker skins have greater amounts of melanin in their skin; this provides more protection against the damaging effects of sunshine.

off at about 24 weeks and replaced by the more complicated double-layered structure of the epidermis and dermis. The function of the periderm is not wholly understood, but it is probably concerned with the absorption of nutrients.

Nails start to take shape 10 weeks after conception. The dermis (mesoderm) develops at 11 weeks, and by 12 weeks indented basal buds of the epidermis form the hair bulbs, with dermal papillae supplying vessels and nerves to the epidermal structures. By 17 weeks, fingerprint ridges are determined and sebaceous glands are becoming active under the influence of maternal hormones that cross the placenta. This sebaceous activity continues until a baby is about six months old, when it peters out, and doesn't kick in again until hormones become active at puberty.

**Between birth and maturity the surface area
of the skin increases sevenfold.**

The teens are often a bad time for skin, but problems are not inevitable and can certainly be treated. Adult skin reflects general health and social behaviour. Anyone who wants their skin to remain relatively soft and unwrinkled until late in life needs to take some precautions: it is vital to avoid excess sun exposure and not to smoke. Ultraviolet light is the cause of almost all the visible changes in sun-exposed areas such as the face and the backs of the hands. Sunblock creams offer partial but not complete protection.

Keeping the skin clean is important to prevent infection and odour, but excess washing can cause dry skin. Washing with harsh soaps strips the skin surface of its natural oils so it's best to choose products with care and avoid having the hands in water for long periods. Similarly, excess washing, colour treating and perming rob the hair of protective oil.

KERATIN: WONDER MATERIAL
The basic protein that makes up the skin, hair and nails is keratin, an amazing substance which forms the major part of the skin and hair, and 98 per cent of the nail plate. Keratin is also found in many other animal species: its toughness and flexibility make it the perfect building block

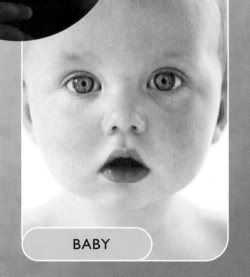

Skin, hair and nail formation
After five months' development a fetus has sweat glands, fine hair on the head, and fully formed eyelids, fingernails and toenails.

PROTECTION FOR LIFE

The resilience of our hair, skin and nails is amazing. For most of us, a modicum of effort in terms of daily maintenance, protection and a good balanced diet will repay us with a lifetime of healthy skin, hair and nails.

BABY

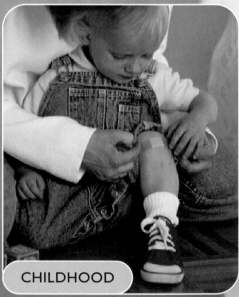

CHILDHOOD

Tender care
A baby's skin is thinner, more fragile and less oily than an adult's. To protect the skin, use baby lotion to seal in moisture after a bath.

Oopsy daisy!
Children regularly fall over, grazing or cutting their skin. At this age the skin heals quickly, but a little antiseptic cream can help prevent infection.

to ensure that birds' feathers fly and horses' hooves are hard. Keratin not only forms the tough substance of the cells, it also creates the anchoring pegs that hold the cells together, side to side and layer upon layer.

There are many different types of keratin in different species and body parts, but they are all made from the same basic amino acid building blocks of cysteine, arginine, lysine and histidine. Cysteine provides the sulphur cross-bonds that link some types of keratin together. These are the bonds that are split by heat or chemicals when a permanent wave is applied to the hair (the bonds reform after the hair cools or the chemicals are neutralised).

The gene sequences which make the different types of keratin have been revealed through research on people in whom keratin production has gone wrong. Some of the most important and life-threatening skin diseases occur when keratin formation is disturbed. Disorders of keratin formation can disrupt the basic structure of the skin: they can make layers of skin slide over each other and let in fluid, causing severe blistering and subsequent infection. Today, skin biopsies can be taken from fetuses known to be at risk of inheriting severe genetic skin disorders – such as Netherton's syndrome and epidermolysis bullosa – at around 16 weeks development.

From boys to men
Teenage boys start to develop facial hair and their skin becomes more oily. In time they will need to start shaving, but each male develops different amounts of body hair.

Sun protection
It is extremely important to protect the skin from sun exposure. Wearing sunscreen, sunglasses and a wide-brimmed hat all help to prevent the ageing effects of UV on the skin.

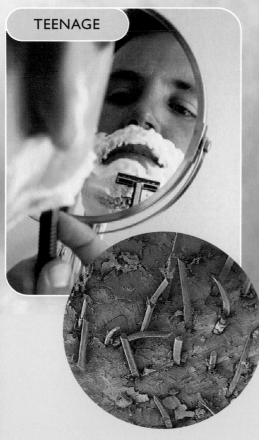

TEENAGE

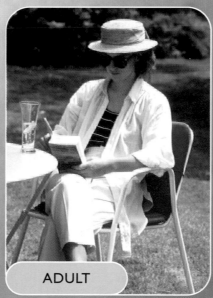

ADULT

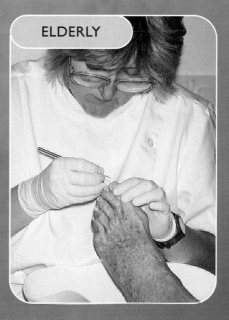

ELDERLY

Keeping skin supple
When stubble hair is shaved, the skin is stripped of its natural oils. After shaving moisturise the skin to prevent dryness.

Foot work
The skin on the feet should receive regular attention. Elderly people often find their mobility is enhanced by chiropody treatment.

The majority of skin diseases are not life-threatening, but rather tend to linger throughout life. Problems such as eczema and psoriasis make up a large proportion of the skin disorders that drive us to seek medical help.

KEEPING UP APPEARANCES

A person's physical appearance is the first thing we notice about them in social situations: 80 per cent of our memory of a person comes from their face – far more than from their voice, and only a minimal amount comes from the content of their conversation. It is no wonder, therefore, that so many of us spend such a lot of our time,

money and effort to make ourselves as attractive as possible to others. In humans the face has evolved to become the most important visual tool, with more than 30 separate muscles involved in controlling facial expression.

Beauty is also a visual impression of form and colour. Appreciation of beauty is subjective, but in any one society there is usually broad agreement on those features which are more – and less – attractive. In our modern society large numbers of individuals are prepared to spend time and money, and even undergo not inconsiderable pain and discomfort, in pursuit of the cultural 'ideal' of beauty.

In the 20th century, the cosmetics industry grew to a multi-million dollar global concern, but efforts to alter the appearance are nothing new. There is evidence of make-up being used in civilisations dating back into antiquity, while tattooing, scarification and piercing have been practised in diverse cultures all over the world for thousands of years. Traditionally, the arts of tattooing and piercing had limited appeal in the West, but they are becoming increasingly popular among groups from all social and economic strata.

Fashions in body adornment constantly shift. At various times in history wigs have been the height of fashion, while at others close-cropped hair has been preferred. Hair colour, length and degree of curl also drift in and out of favour. One of the earliest uses of make-up was to make warriors more fearsome to their opponents, but it soon became a way to enhance attractiveness. It has been used to produce the 'pale and interesting' look considered desirable in much of the past, but this has given way to the era of the suntan – still with us despite escalating evidence of its harmful effects on the skin.

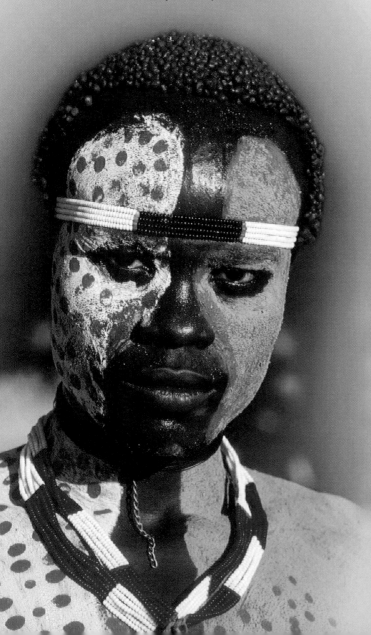

Identity art
Throughout history, skin decoration and body art has been of deep significance in cultures around the world. It has been used to provide a link to ancestors, to convey religious symbolism, to mark rites of passage and to emphasise visual characteristics.

SKIN COLOUR

A number of factors influence our skin colour. Genetics plays a major part, as does geographical region and the amount of time spent outdoors. Other factors include haemoglobin, internally produced pigments such as bilirubin, and the amounts of melanin and phaeomelanin in the skin and hair. In many conditions temporary or permanent changes can occur to skin and hair colour which can lead to distress and even psychological illness.

Skin colour can be a major factor in all sorts of prejudices, and not just between races of different colour. Departures from the norm in a society can have unhappy consequences for individuals and their place within society.

SKIN IN THE FUTURE

The global loss of protective ozone over the past 20 years means that we are being exposed to more UV radiation than previous generations, even though most of us are more 'sun aware'. UV damage initially causes fine lines on the skin, but repeated sun exposure eventually makes deep wrinkles and may result in skin cancer. Estimates suggest that a 1 per cent decrease in ozone can result in a 5 per cent increase in skin cancer rates: ozone depletion may increase our children's risk of skin cancer by up to 15 per cent, making vigilance in skin protection evermore vital.

On a more positive note for the future, scientists have succeeded in culturing epidermal skin from a tiny undamaged area of human skin. This has major implications for severe burns victims, greatly increasing their chances of survival and minimising eventual scarring. Parallel to this has been the development of artificial skin, a non-living material free from bacteria and viruses. Artificial skin is used to support the grafted epidermis, which then

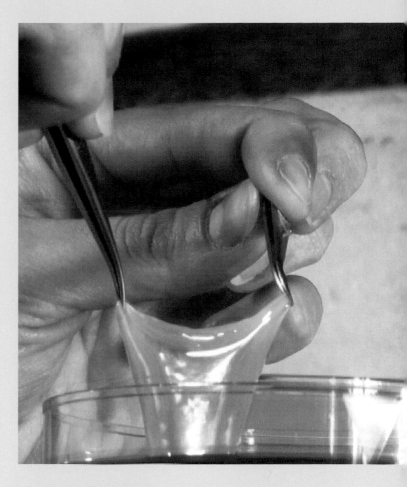

Sample of artificial skin
Scientific advances have led to the development of artificially grown skin. Its three layers – epidermis, dermis and hypodermis – have all the specialised cells and structures found in normal skin.

regenerates the dermal layer. The world's first factory making human skin opened in 1995. Researchers are also looking at the genetics involved in baldness and greying hair with a view to modifying the genes responsible to prevent both processes. In the not too distant future, gene therapy may also be the key to successful treatment of melanoma.

There are reputed to be more than 2000 skin conditions, but two-thirds of skin diseases are caused by fewer than 10 conditions. Skin problems account for 10 per cent of all GP consultations in the UK.

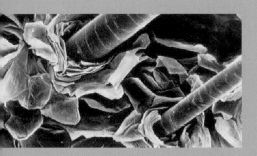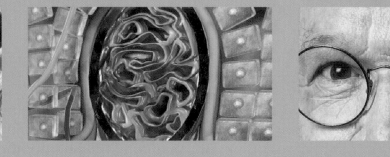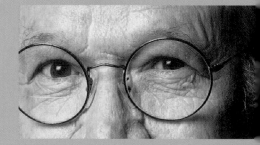

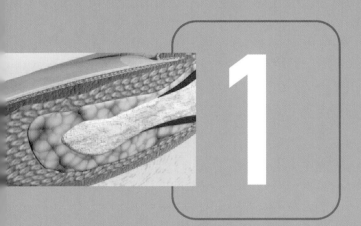

1

How your skin, hair and nails work

Your amazing skin, hair and nails

Your skin is the largest and most versatile system of tissue organisation that you have. As a barrier between you and the outside world it fulfills many roles, starting with keeping water out and your insides safely covered.

The skin is the largest organ in the body, weighing on average 4kg (9 pounds) and covering a surface area of about 2 square metres (2.5 square yards).

WHY DO WE NEED SKIN?

The skin – the outer covering of the body – has several extremely important functions. It protects you from water loss and damage from ultraviolet radiation. It helps you to regulate your body temperature. It is an effective barrier against injury and invading microorganisms, and it is involved in the immune response that protects the body from foreign substances that do manage to penetrate it. Nerve impulses from the skin communicate sensation to the brain. The skin plays an essential part in the production of vitamin D – vital for healthy bones. In addition, it has a role in display and sexual attraction.

THE CHANGING FACE OF SKIN

Although the basic structure of the skin is the same over the entire body, there are local variations linked to differences in function. For example, the skin on the palms of the hands and soles of the feet has no hair, and is much thicker than in other areas in order to toughen it up. Skin regularly exposed to sunlight is darker than skin hidden from view to help protect it from ultraviolet radiation.

The appearance of the skin varies throughout life, and even day-to-day changes can occur, depending on your emotions and state of well-being: skin abnormalities can often be the first warning of internal illness.

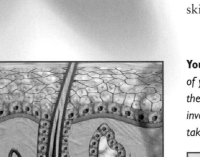

Your nails protect *protect the sensitive tips of your fingers and toes from damage, and they also form valuable tools for tasks involving prising or scratching. Pages 32–33 take a close-up look at these appendages.*

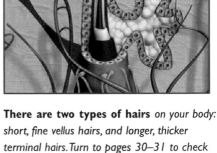

There are two types of hairs *on your body: short, fine vellus hairs, and longer, thicker terminal hairs. Turn to pages 30–31 to check out their differences – and find out why some vellus hairs turn into terminal hairs at puberty.*

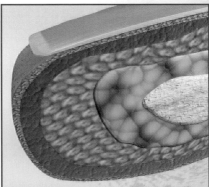

Tiny blood vessels *in the dermis not only nourish the skin and aid in combating infection by bringing in white blood cells, but also help the body to cool off or warm up as required. Pages 26–27 describe how.*

16

Hair, nails and glands
*Parts of your epidermis have become
specialised and form the so-called
epidermal appendages, which project
deep into the dermis. These are the
hairs and nails, the sebaceous glands
and the sweat glands.*

A sweat gland *is a long, coiled, hollow
tube that transports sweat to the skin's
surface so it can evaporate. To find out
more about how the body stays cool,
turn to pages 26–27.*

Each strand of hair *extends 4–5mm
into the skin's subterranean layers. To
find out more, see pages 30–31.*

The epidermis *is the outermost layer of the
skin. The dead skin cells are continually shed and
replaced from the cell layers beneath. Find out
how and why this happens on pages 18–19.*

**Sensory nerve
endings** *in the
dermis provide you
with your sense of
touch – one of the
five key senses. Find
out more on
pages 22–23.*

A sebaceous gland
*produces sebum that
lubricates, protects and
waterproofs the skin.
Find out more about
this wonder fluid on
pages 24–25.*

The dermis *is the layer of connective
tissue beneath the epidermis that
forms the bulk of the skin. Discover
more about its crucial supporting
role on pages 20–21.*

The structure of the skin
*The skin is made up of two layers, the
epidermis and the dermis. The topmost level
of the epidermis is a tough protective layer of
dead cells that rub off constantly as they are
replaced by cells moving up from below.
Beneath the dermis is a deep layer of
subcutaneous fat.*

Layer of subcutaneous fat

The epidermis

The epidermis is a multi-layered, self-renewing structure that varies in thickness from less than a tenth of a millimetre on the eyelids to nearly one millimetre on the palms of the hands and soles of the feet.

GOING UP!

The epidermis renews itself constantly by cell division at its deepest layer, the basal layer. Keratinocyte cells produced by division in the basal layer are pushed upwards towards the surface to become, in turn, the prickle cell layer, the granular layer and – last of all – the horny layer, also called the stratum corneum, where they die. As the cells ascend towards the surface they alter in structure and function. The time it takes for cells to pass from the basal cell layer to the horny layer is about 14 days. Then it takes another 14 days or so for cells in the horny layer to die and be rubbed off by daily wear and tear.

The epidermis varies in depth from five cells to thirty cells, depending on the part of the body. The thickness of the skin at any one part of the body always remains constant: the cells lost at the skin surface are balanced by new skin cells produced in the basal layer. Complex systems of cell growth regulation come into action to speed up or slow down cell division and maturation in the epidermis.

4 **The horny layer** (stratum corneum) sits above the granular layer. By now the cells are flattened, with no nuclei or granules. The cells of the horny layer overlap each other like tiles, with the edges stuck together with a fatty 'cement' ideal for waterproofing purposes. The horny layer varies in thickness according to the region of the body; it is thickest on the soles of the feet.

3 **The granular layer** is made up of flattened keratinocytes that contain not only granules of the protein keratohyalin but also lamellar granules that produce a 'cement' which binds the cells together.

2 **The prickle cell layer** is composed mainly of keratinocytes packed closely together.

1 **The basal layer cells** are shaped like upturned bricks. They are anchored to a basement membrane, from which threads extend down to anchor the membrane to the upper dermis.

Melanocytes

Interspersed among the basal cells are the melanocytes, adapted nerve tissue cells that send out projections called dendrites between the epidermal cells. They produce the melanin that gives skin its colour (see pages 28–29).

Merkel cells

These cells are concentrated in areas around hair follicles in the basal layer, and probably transmit the sensation of light touch to the brain. Other nerve endings in the skin are sensitive to deeper pressure and temperature changes.

Inside view
*Here, the very top covering of
the horny layer of the epidermis
has been peeled back, revealing
the pattern of the flattened
cells beneath.*

*Approximately
30,000 dead skin cells
are shed from the
epidermis every minute.*

KERATIN – WONDER SUBSTANCE
The epidermis is largely made up of keratin
– a protein that in effect provides the body
with a protective coating. It is keratin that
prevents too much moisture evaporating
from the surface of the skin. Keratin is
virtually impenetrable to harmful
substances, and also has anti-bacterial
properties. Keratin is also a major
constituent of the epidermal appendages,
the hair and nails.

Keratinocytes
Ninety-five per cent of all cells in the epidermis are
keratinocytes – these are the cells that slowly move upwards
from the basal layer to the skin's surface. They contain
keratin – the main structural protein of the epidermis.
Threads of keratin within keratinocytes in the basal and
prickle cell layers gradually combine to form bundles
which interweave and then become stuck together by a
'cement' produced by granules in the granular layer. By the
time they reach the horny layer they form a mat that is an
almost impenetrable barrier stopping substances from passing
in and out of the body.

Langerhans cells
These are found in the prickle cell layer and, like
melanocytes, they are dendritic cells. The first
line of defence against environmental hazards,
they seize harmful microorganisms and
deliver them to lymphocytes in the dermis, so
that an immune response can be generated.

19

The dermis

The dermis is the layer of connective tissue that lies between the epidermis above and the subcutaneous fat below. Its function is to support the epidermis structurally and nutritionally.

HOLDING IT ALL TOGETHER

The dermis is a network of interwoven fibres, composed principally of collagen and including a significant amount of elastin, which gives the skin its great strength and elasticity. These fibres are embedded in a strong ground substance of complex carbohydrates – mucopolysaccharides – that act as structural components in the connective tissue. Also within the dermis are several different types of cell – fibroblasts, mast cells and macrophages – each with a different function. In addition, the dermis contains blood vessels, lymphatic vessels, nerves and muscles. Nerve endings in the dermis act as receptors that pick up the sensations of light and heavy touch, pain, heat and cold.

Macrophages *are a type of phagocyte. Their job is to consume cellular waste material and other debris, including bacteria.*

The thickness of the dermis varies from 3mm or more on the soles of the feet to just 0.6mm in the eyelids.

Merkel cell

Collagen *is the predominant fibre in the dermis. It is packed into bundles to give the skin strength and prevent tearing. Elastic fibres mingled with the collagen help the skin to return to its original shape after movement or injury.*

Sweat gland

Fibroblasts *make up the majority of the cells in the dermis. They produce the connective tissue that 'knits' the dermis together. They tend to be located near collagen and elastin fibres.*

Subcutaneous fat layer

Blood vessels *in the skin help with temperature regulation. The network of vessels just above the subcutaneous fat also supplies the sweat glands and hair follicles.*

**Basal layer of
the epidermis**

The ground substance *of the dermis is a semi-solid gel
in which fibres and cells are embedded. It holds water
but allows nutrients, hormones and waste products to
pass through. It lubricates the collagen and elastin fibres
when the skin moves. It also provides bulk, allowing the
dermis to act as a shock absorber.*

**A basement
membrane** *separates the
epidermis and
dermis.*

**A Meissner's
corpuscle** *is a type
of touch receptor.*

Mast cells *are specialised cells that spring
into action when challenged by external injury
or foreign substances. Granules inside each cell
release histamine and other chemicals that
play an important role in the inflammatory
response to infection.*

Lymphocytes *are white blood
cells involved in protecting the
body from infection. They move
between the lymphatic system
and the bloodstream.*

Pacinian corpuscles
*are one of several kinds
of touch receptor found
in the dermis – see*
pages 22–23.

SUBCUTANEOUS FAT
The subcutaneous fat layer that
sits below the dermis separates
the skin from underlying bones
and muscles. It is made up of
loose connective tissue
intermingled with fat cells. Its
thickness varies, depending on
its location within the body.
The boundary between the
dermis and subcutaneous layer
is generally indistinct; the one
merges into the other.

Touch

The skin is packed with sensory receptors that give your body its sense of touch. This provides the brain with vital clues about the body in relation to its environment, so it can act accordingly, as when withdrawing fingers from heat, for instance.

MAKING SENSE OF YOUR ENVIRONMENT

Sensory receptors within the epidermis and dermis can pick up touch, pain, heat and cold. Sensory nerves vary in complexity, but all react to physical sensations, converting them into nerve impulses that are transmitted along the central nervous system to the thalamus inside the brain. In the thalamus, these impulses are identified and relayed to the appropriate sensory regions of the brain. Every second, billions of signals are transmitted to the brain from stimuli all over the body, and processed to create a sensory image and warn of any danger. The sensory receptor cells that lie within the epidermis or the upper dermis tend to be very sensitive to touch and heat; others, located deeper within the dermis, specialise in detecting heavier pressure.

Touch receptors

Touch receptors are types of sensory receptors. They range from free nerve endings to more complex tactile receptors enclosed in capsules of connective tissue. There are touch receptors all over the body, but some areas of skin – notably the palms, soles and lips – have more than others and as a result are more sensitive to touch and pain.

Sensation and communication

Touching the skin has great psychological importance: stroking and cuddling promotes emotional development, learning and growth in newborn infants, while touching is known to enhance emotional well-being in people of all ages. Parts of the skin are also considered to be erogenous zones.

The skin has around a million nerve endings; most of these are in the skin on the face and hands, with relatively few on the back.

Epidermis

Blood vessels

Free nerve endings *are widespread all over the upper part of the dermis. They protrude into the epidermis.*

Dermis

Merkel's discs *sense continuous light touch and pressure against the skin. Unlike other touch receptors, they are not covered by a capsule of connective tissue.*

Meissner's corpuscles *are especially sensitive touch receptors that are found in the upper dermis of the fingertips and palms, the lips, the soles of the feet, eyelids, nipples and external genitalia.*

Ruffini's corpuscles *are touch receptors located deeper in the dermis; they pick up heavy prolonged touch and pressure.*

Pacinian corpuscles *detect the rapid movement (vibration) of tissues and changes in pressure; they are found deep in the dermis, also close to muscles and joints, and in the wall of the bladder.*

23

Protecting the body

The skin protects the body from the environment and from infection. Various mechanisms come into play to ensure that this protection is effective.

A BARRIER TO INFECTION

The skin's first line of defence is its robust, protective outer layer. Keratin, collagen and elastin combine to form a tough but flexible covering. Sebum helps to keep the skin supple. Pigment in skin protects against ultraviolet radiation by absorbing and scattering the rays and by scavenging free radicals. In addition, the dryness and constant shedding of dead skin cells, benign microorganisms (mostly bacteria) that normally live on the skin, the fatty acids of sebum and the lactic acid of sweat, all combine to repel invading bacteria, viruses, fungi and parasites. Langherhans' cells in the epidermis and lymphoid tissue also play an active role in monitoring the skin for foreign substances and particles, acting quickly to eliminate them.

How invaders breach the skin

Despite these protective measures, infectious organisms can enter the skin in various ways. Natural openings abound: sweat pores, hair follicles and sebaceous gland openings all allow bacteria, viruses and fungal infections to enter. Broken skin or insect bites can be the port of entry for disease, such as malaria. Warm, moist areas are prone to fungal infections such as athlete's foot.

Hair shaft

Horny layer of the skin – the stratum corneum

Sebum – an oily coating that cleans and seals

- Sebaceous glands are located on the skin wherever there are hair follicles. They are larger and more numerous on the scalp, face, chest and back. Most open into hair follicles; the only exceptions to these are sebaceous glands on the eyelids, in the genital area and on the nipples.
- The sebum secreted by sebaceous glands is an oily compound containing various fatty substances. It enables the skin's outermost layer to retain water, and controls water loss from the epidermis. The free fatty acids in sebum act as a disinfectant, helping to prevent bacteria and fungi from colonising the skin.
- Sebum is produced at birth in response to maternal hormones, then disappears until puberty when sebaceous glands develop, stimulated by androgens (the hormones produced by the testis), adrenal glands and – to a lesser extent – the ovaries in women.

Sebum on the skin

Sebum within a sebaceous gland

Dermis

Touch receptor

Hair follicle

Subcutaneous fat layer

A waterproof jacket
- *If you had no horny outer layer of the skin, you would lose significant amounts of water to the environment and become dehydrated. The lipid bilayer, a fine layer of fats on the outer surface of the horny layer, stops water evaporating from the skin and makes it very difficult for water to enter from outside.*
- *There are times when the skin's ability to keep out water can become slightly impaired. This may happen when the horny layer is excessively dry or soggy, warmer than usual, or damaged in some way – perhaps by a detergent. Scientists take these factors into account when developing drug delivery systems, or formulating cosmetic face creams.*

Sweat expelled onto the skin

Epidermis

Eccrine sweat gland

Blood vessel

White blood cells *move towards a site of infection.*

The inflammatory response – localising the damage
- *If foreign organisms do penetrate the body's protective defence barriers, the body's response is to generate inflammation of the immediate area, to prevent infection becoming more widespread.*
- *The damaged tissue releases chemicals that attract specialised scavenging cells – phagocyte-type white blood cells – to the infected area. Blood vessels inside the dermis dilate, increasing blood flow to the area. The walls of these tiny blood vessels become porous, allowing the phagocytes to move from the blood vessel into the area of tissue damage, where they engulf and destroy the invading microorganisms.*
- *The characteristic red, swollen, hot appearance of inflamed tissue is caused by the swollen blood vessels and the sharp increase in the number of cells in the tissue. The affected area becomes painful when the chemicals released during this process – such as serotonin and histamine – stimulate nerve endings in the dermis.*

Regulating temperature

Humans do not have a thick fur coat to provide warmth. Instead we rely on a complex system of specialised blood vessels in the skin and the action of the sweat glands to regulate heat loss and conservation.

WHEN THE BODY IS TOO HOT

When the temperature of the body increases and needs to be brought down again, the blood vessels near the surface of the skin dilate. This allows more blood to reach the skin, so that heat is lost and the blood cools down. This brings a flushed appearance to the skin. How much the blood vessels dilate is controlled by nerves known as vasomotor fibres, which are controlled by the brain.

At the same time, eccrine sweat glands produce increased amounts of sweat, which evaporates on the surface of the skin to cool the skin. When the air is dry, the sweating mechanism is a very effective way of maintaining a tolerable body temperature. But in humid heat, when sweat cannot evaporate so easily, the sweating mechanism is not so helpful and the body may overheat.

WHEN THE BODY IS TOO COLD

If the body is too cold, the blood vessels close to the surface of the skin constrict to reduce the flow of blood. Warm blood is diverted into deeper blood vessels and so heat is conserved (and the skin becomes paler).

The layer of subcutaneous fat under the dermis provides extra insulation and, in addition, the arrector pili muscles – the tiny muscles attached to hair follicles – contract, lifting the hairs until they become erect. This has the effect of pulling on the skin to produce goose bumps. In mammals with long, thick hair, the erect hairs trap a layer of warm air at the skin's surface; in humans this only has a small effect because human body hair is so short and fine. Fear and anger also make body hair stand on end.

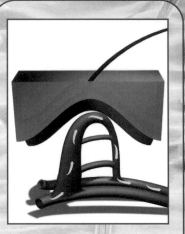

Cooling down when too hot
The tiny blood vessels close to the skin's surface expand to increase the surface area of the blood vessel walls, so that more heat can escape from the blood passing through.

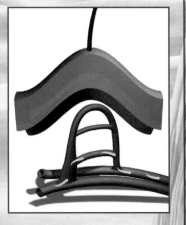

Conserving heat when too cold
The tiny blood vessels near the skin's surface contract to reduce the amount of surface area from which heat can escape from the blood in the vessels.

There are about two-and-a-half million sweat glands on the surface of your skin.

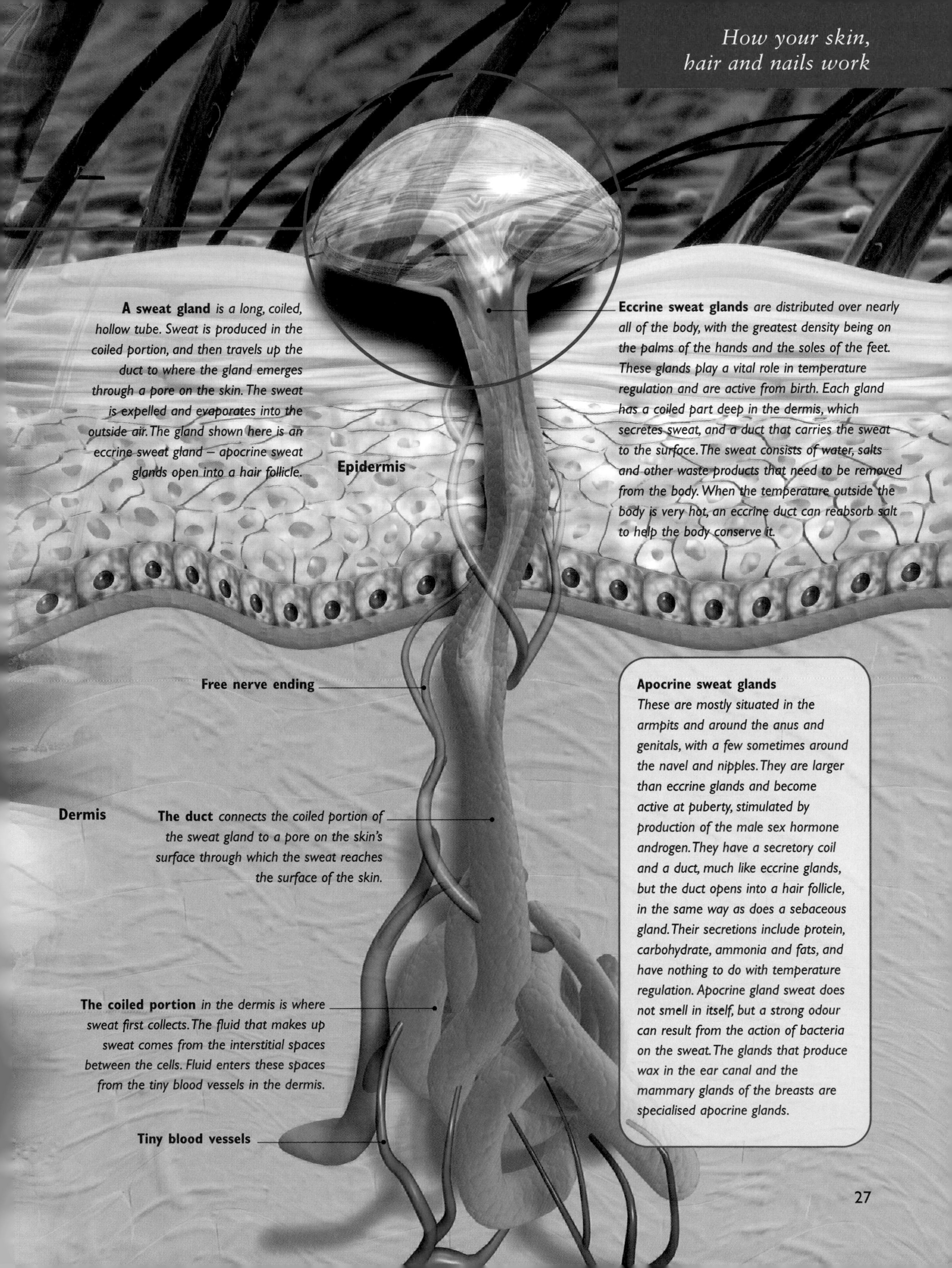

A sweat gland *is a long, coiled, hollow tube. Sweat is produced in the coiled portion, and then travels up the duct to where the gland emerges through a pore on the skin. The sweat is expelled and evaporates into the outside air. The gland shown here is an eccrine sweat gland — apocrine sweat glands open into a hair follicle.*

Epidermis

Eccrine sweat glands *are distributed over nearly all of the body, with the greatest density being on the palms of the hands and the soles of the feet. These glands play a vital role in temperature regulation and are active from birth. Each gland has a coiled part deep in the dermis, which secretes sweat, and a duct that carries the sweat to the surface. The sweat consists of water, salts and other waste products that need to be removed from the body. When the temperature outside the body is very hot, an eccrine duct can reabsorb salt to help the body conserve it.*

Free nerve ending

Dermis

The duct *connects the coiled portion of the sweat gland to a pore on the skin's surface through which the sweat reaches the surface of the skin.*

Apocrine sweat glands
These are mostly situated in the armpits and around the anus and genitals, with a few sometimes around the navel and nipples. They are larger than eccrine glands and become active at puberty, stimulated by production of the male sex hormone androgen. They have a secretory coil and a duct, much like eccrine glands, but the duct opens into a hair follicle, in the same way as does a sebaceous gland. Their secretions include protein, carbohydrate, ammonia and fats, and have nothing to do with temperature regulation. Apocrine gland sweat does not smell in itself, but a strong odour can result from the action of bacteria on the sweat. The glands that produce wax in the ear canal and the mammary glands of the breasts are specialised apocrine glands.

The coiled portion *in the dermis is where sweat first collects. The fluid that makes up sweat comes from the interstitial spaces between the cells. Fluid enters these spaces from the tiny blood vessels in the dermis.*

Tiny blood vessels

The colour of skin and hair

Compared with many creatures from the animal kingdom, humans have a rather limited colour palette when it comes to skin and hair – we largely rely on shades of brown and red.

FROM BLACK TO WHITE

Brown skin – and hair – coloration is due to melanin, with the intensity of colour varying from almost white (no melanin) to almost jet black (a large amount). The amount of melanin our skin and hair contains is determined genetically.

MELANIN

Melanin is a pigment produced by specialised cells called melanocytes. These are found in the basal layer of the epidermis. Each melanocyte contains melanosomes, in which melanin is synthesised. These melanosomes are engulfed by keratinocyte cells and it is differences in their behaviour here that determine skin colour.

There are also melanocytes in the bulbs of hair follicles (and in the retina of the eye). Melanocytes in a hair bulb are packaged into granules that pigment the hair shaft.

Hair colour
Melanin produces a limited colour palette in hair: shades of yellow, brown, red and black.
Two forms of melanin colour hair:

- *Eumelanin is the dark pigment which predominates in black and brunette hair. Phaeomelanin is lighter and found in red and blonde hair. Many people's hair contains a mixture of the two: the more phaeomelanin, the lighter the hair.*
- *The combination of pigments in any one head of hair is determined genetically. People of Celtic origin tend to have more phaeomelanin than people of other races: hence the classic combination of red hair and very pale skin.*
- *The age at which hair starts to turn grey is also genetically determined. This occurs as production of the melanin that colours the hair slowly decreases and the cells in the medulla at the centre of each terminal hair shaft become filled instead with tiny air bubbles that reflect light. It is because of the way that hairs without melanin reflect light that they appear to be white.*

In pale-skinned people
melanosomes are clustered together in melanosome complexes that gradually degenerate as the skin cells rise towards the surface.

MELANIN AND SUN EXPOSURE

Melanin helps to protect the skin from damage caused by ultraviolet radiation (UVR) from the sun, by absorbing the UVR before it penetrates to deeper layers of the epidermis and dermis. UVR is, however, useful for helping to produce vitamin D – important for calcium metabolism and strong, healthy bones – and so a moderate amount of UVR on the skin is beneficial, especially for people whose diet is deficient in this vitamin.

Getting a suntan

Sunbathing leads to a suntan through two processes, one immediate and one taking place over the next few days. First, UVR (mainly UVA) darkens the skin by oxidising melanin that already exists; UVB stimulates the melanocytes to produce more melanin. The reason that some people tan more easily than others is because these people have melanocytes in their skin that are more active.

An evolutionary puzzle
Why do people have different coloured skins, which seem to be related to the part of the world from which they originate? The main reason is to protect them from sun damage: people in hotter countries have melanocytes in their skin that are more active and produce more melanin to absorb the potentially damaging UVR from the sun. Also, it has been postulated that having a paler skin enables more UVR absorption and therefore enhances vitamin D production for people living in regions of the world with less reliable sunshine.

Horny topmost layer of the epidermis

Granular layer of the epidermis

Prickle cell layer of the epidermis

Melanosomes containing melanin *travel along the tentacle-like dendrites of each melanocyte. From here they transfer to the keratinocytes that surround them.*

Keratinocyte

A melanocyte *with nucleus surrounded by cell membranes. Melanocytes are found in the basal cell layer of the epidermis, just above the dermis. They produce and store melanosomes.*

Basal layer of the epidermis

In people born with darker skins *the melanosomes are greater in number and larger in size; they stay separate and they remain active as they migrate upwards, breaking down less rapidly than in people with paler skins.*

Basement membrane

Dermis

All about hair

Virtually the whole of the surface of your skin is covered with hairs – be they obvious or not. The only hair-free zones are the palms of the hands, the soles of the feet, the nipples, the lips and the eyelids.

HAIR TYPES

Hair is made of the protein keratin that also makes up your nails and is a major constituent of the epidermis. There are two main types of hair.

- **Vellus hairs** are the short, fine, usually light-coloured hairs that cover most of the body's surface. Vellus hairs on the body can change into terminal hairs in hirsutism, a condition of excessive hair growth.
- **Terminal hairs** are the longer, thicker, generally darker hairs that appear on the scalp, in the eyebrows and eyelashes, and in the armpits and genital area. Some groups of terminal hairs begin life as vellus hairs but change under the influence of hormones at puberty. These include the hair in the armpits and genital area, some leg hair, and men also develop a beard and more body hair. When a man begins to lose the hair on his scalp, this reflects terminal hairs changing into vellus hairs.

WHAT IS HAIR FOR?

Most of the hair on your body performs no vital function – you could be hairless without any significant disturbance to your body's equilibrium. Some hair does have a practical function, however: eyelashes protect the eyes from foreign particles; eyebrows direct sweat away from the eyes; hair on the scalp protects the head from ultraviolet radiation. Erect vellus hairs help to conserve heat within the body when temperatures drop (see pages 26–27).

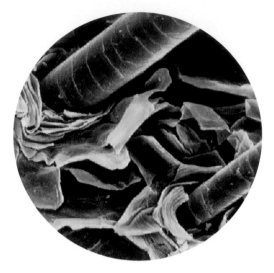

What makes hairs straight or curly?
In this coloured electron micrograph of hair shafts protruding from a scalp, the roundness of each hair shaft indicates that these are straight hairs. The rounder the cross-section of the shaft, the straighter the hair will be; the flatter the cross-section, the more the hair will curl.

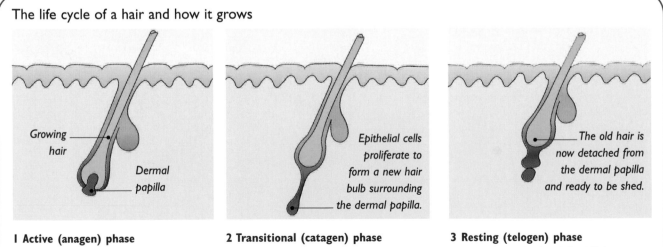

The life cycle of a hair and how it grows

Growing hair

Dermal papilla

Epithelial cells proliferate to form a new hair bulb surrounding the dermal papilla.

The old hair is now detached from the dermal papilla and ready to be shed.

1 Active (anagen) phase
This is the period during which the hair shaft grows. The active phase lasts from two to five years for hair on the scalp.

2 Transitional (catagen) phase
This is a short resting period after the hair has stopped growing. On the scalp this phase lasts about two weeks.

3 Resting (telogen) phase
The old hair is shed and the follicle prepares for a new hair shaft. On the scalp this phase lasts for three or four months.

The cuticle *of a hair is made up of a thin layer of cells containing keratin. They overlap each other in a similar way to roof tiles, with the free margins pointing towards the tip of the hair. A 'split end' may result if this layer wears away.*

The hair shaft *is the part of a hair that is visible above the surface of the skin.*

Epidermis

The cortex *consists of packed keratinocytes and contains the melanin pigment that gives the hair its colour.*

The hair follicle *is beneath the skin's surface. It is a specialised tubular construction of epidermal cells that grows down into the dermis at an angle and contains the hair root.*

In the medulla, *at the centre of a terminal hair, cells intermingle with air spaces. In vellus hairs there is no medulla at all.*

Basement membrane

There is a sebaceous gland *associated with each hair follicle. It helps to lubricate the hair.*

Outer root sheath

Dermis

An arrector pili muscle *is attached to each hair follicle. When this bundle of muscle fibres contracts, the hair is pulled upright, creating a 'goose bump'.*

Sensory nerve endings

The hair bulb *at the lower end of the follicle encloses the dermal papilla. Included within the hair bulb are melanocytes and keratinocytes that give the hair its colour and texture.*

The dermal papilla *contains dividing cells, and receives blood vessels and nerve endings that nourish the growing hair. It is from the dermal papilla that a new hair grows once the old hair has died.*

The ends of the line

As our principal instruments of touch, the fingertips are in constant use and, along with the vulnerable toes, are in need of extra protection. This is provided by the nails, which on the fingers also make useful tools in themselves.

The skin on the fingertips is particularly well supplied with nerve endings. Each fingertip has more than 3000 touch receptors.

THE NAILS

The nail is, in fact, the evolutionary remnant of a mammalian claw. It consists of a plate of hardened and densely packed keratin. In addition to protecting the finger ends, the nails have valuable prising and picking skills.

How fast do nails grow?

The rate at which nails grow varies from person to person. Fingernails grow continuously and average between 0.5 and 1.2mm per week. Toenails grow about a third more slowly. Nails grow faster when you are younger, and faster in summertime than in winter, possibly because blood circulates at a faster rate in summer, triggering more rapid cell division. It takes about six months for a fingernail to grow from the matrix to the free edge, and up to 18 months for the nail on the big toe to do the same. The nails on your dominant hand grow a little faster than those on your non-dominant hand. Diseases of the nail, skin or body can affect the growth rate of the nails generally. Nails do not continue to grow for a short time after death, as is sometimes thought, but the nail folds do shrink away from the nail plate, creating the illusion that the nail has grown.

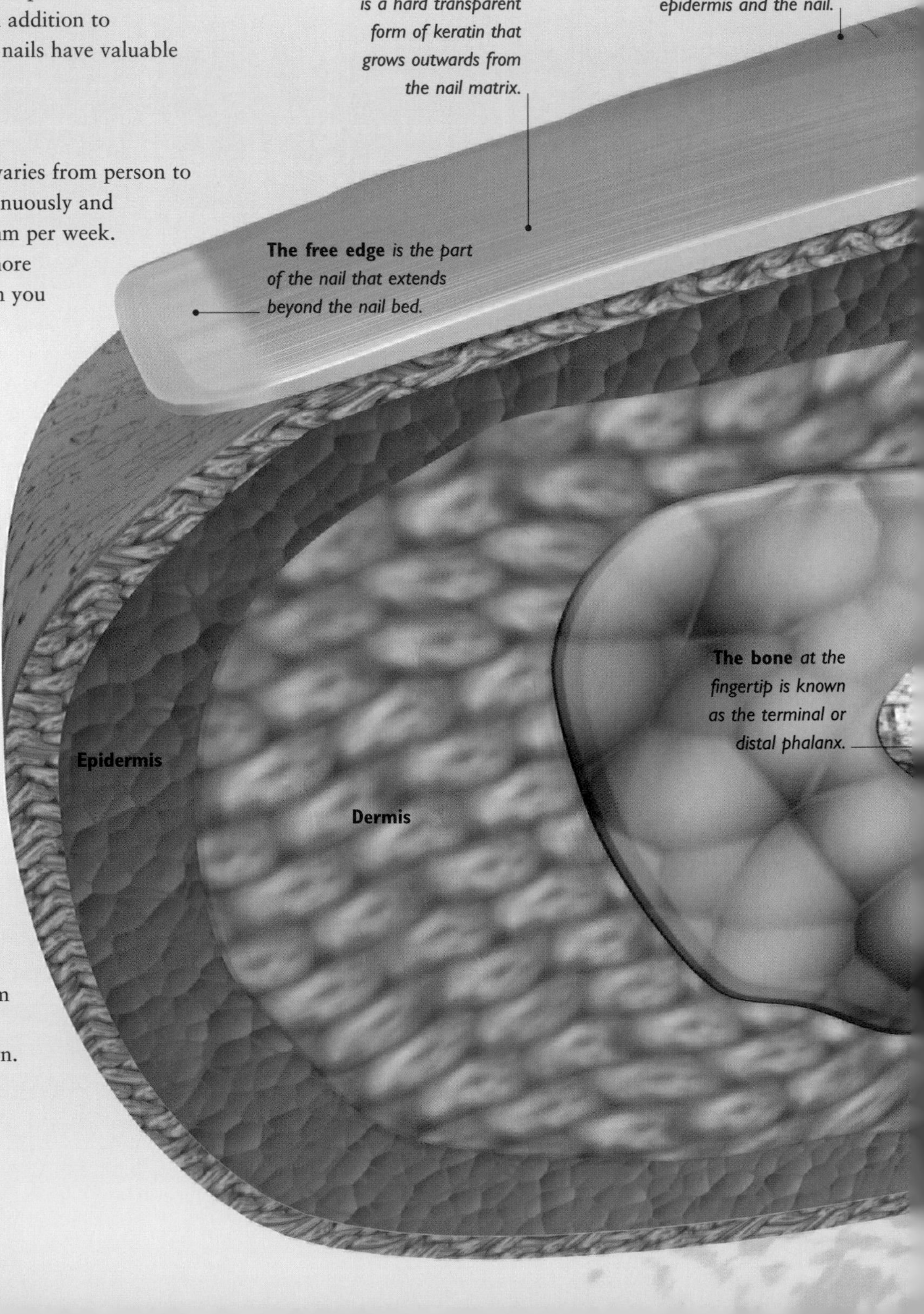

The lateral nail fold is the bulge of skin on either side of the nail, at the boundary of the epidermis and the nail.

The nail plate is a hard transparent form of keratin that grows outwards from the nail matrix.

The free edge is the part of the nail that extends beyond the nail bed.

The bone at the fingertip is known as the terminal or distal phalanx.

Epidermis

Dermis

The lunula *is the only part of the matrix that you can see. It looks like a pale 'half-moon' at the base of the nail plate (lunula is Latin for 'crescent-shaped moon').*

The cuticle *is an extension of the horny layer of the skin of the nail fold. It acts as a seal to protect the matrix from infection.*

Proximal nail fold

The nail bed *lies immediately beneath the nail plate.*

A layer of fat *surrounds the bone at the end of the finger.*

The matrix or root of the nail *runs from the proximal nail fold to the outer edge of the lunula. From this root, the nail plate grows over the nail bed, ending in a free edge at the fingertip. It is in the matrix that keratin is produced, by cell division. Therefore, if the matrix is destroyed the nail can't grow back.*

WHAT IS A FINGERPRINT?

On the fingertips the outermost layer of skin forms tiny ridges that make up the distinctive patterns that we call our fingerprints. These ridges are found all over the palms of the hands and the soles of the feet. The patterns they form are unique to you (only identical twins share the same patterns). The ridges follow the same patterns that are created below the skin's surface, where the dermis and epidermis join by means of interlocking projections down from the epidermis (called rete ridges) and up from the dermis (dermal papillae). The projections lock the dermis and epidermis together.

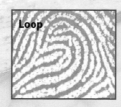
Loop

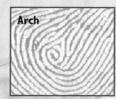
Arch

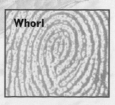
Whorl

Distinctive patterns
Loops are the most common fingertip ridge patterns; arches are the least common. Everyone has a unique pattern of loops, whorls and arches.

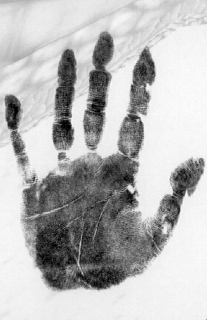

A lifetime of skin, hair and nails

From birth through adolescence to middle age and beyond, your skin and hair slowly change in appearance. These changes are mostly due to the natural maturing and ageing processes – but the effects of too much sun exposure can also become apparent as the years go by.

SMOOTH AS SILK?

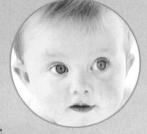

A baby's skin is often hailed as being perfect, but for newborns this may be far from the case. In general a baby's skin is thinner, less oily and more fragile than that of an adult, so it becomes irritated, sore and sunburnt more easily. Prominent sebaceous glands or whitish bumps may appear; both should disappear naturally in a few weeks. Babies don't sweat as efficiently as adults, and sometimes little blisters caused by blocked sweat ducts can develop.

A baby's hair is usually very fine and babies are frequently born blond, developing darker hair as they become older. A premature baby may be born with fine, long hairs – called lanugo hairs – covering the head, shoulders and back. These form in the fetus at around 20 weeks, but they are normally shed before a birth that is full-term.

Babies are born with soft, rapidly growing nails that are almost always perfect – congenital abnormalities of the nails are very rare.

TEENAGE TRAUMA

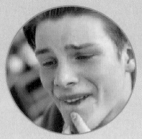

The hormone testosterone begins to be produced in both sexes, causing the sebaceous glands in hair follicles and pores to produce the natural oil known as sebum. When the body overproduces sebum, dead skin cells tend to clog the sebaceous glands, creating the blemishes that characterise acne. Sebaceous gland activity can also make hair more greasy. Hormones also trigger the conversion of vellus hairs in the genital areas and armpits into terminal hairs – as well as the growth of facial hair and more terminal body hair in adolescent boys.

THE MIDDLE YEARS

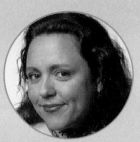

In the middle years, the dermis begins to hold less water and fat so that skin loses its 'roundness' and starts to sag. The skin becomes less resilient, as fewer elastic fibres are produced. It becomes dryer in response to less sebum being produced and cell renewal takes longer, so older cells remain on the skin surface longer, causing creases and wrinkles. This process is apparent in most people by their late 40s; in those who have spent time in the sun or who smoke, it becomes apparent earlier.

Hair begins to turn grey and some men start to lose their hair. The age at which this happens is genetically determined, but, like the skin, hair is also affected by ultraviolet radiation (UVR) from the sun, becoming dry and coarse after a lot of sun exposure.

As the body gets older, the nails harden, particularly the toenails, and life starts to take its toll on the feet and nails, with problems such as hard skin developing.

SIGNS OF LIFE

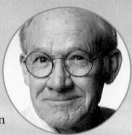

As the body ages, the skin becomes progressively thinner and more wrinkled due to loss of elasticity, collagen, moisture and fat. Exposure to UVR speeds up this ageing process, especially in Caucasian skin. In addition, the number of melanocytes (which contain the pigment melanin) in the skin gradually decrease with advancing age, making skin even more susceptible to UVR damage, and so also to skin cancer.

With advancing years the amount of sebum produced falls (slightly in men, significantly in women) so that skin becomes dryer and less supple. The amount of collagen in the skin decreases by about 1 per cent per year through adult life, more in women after the menopause, causing skin to sag. Fewer fibroblasts are present in the dermis, meaning that wounds heal more slowly. Over the age of 70, the skin is less able to regulate body heat, which is why the elderly are so much more susceptible to the effects of severe cold weather.

A day in the life of the skin and hair

It's the weekend and you have the opportunity to spend time with family and friends, and take things at a more leisurely pace than normal. Your skin and hair, however, cannot take a break from their work of protecting you from the outside world.

SKIN CONSCIOUS

Your skin is constantly working to keep you well. It helps to cool you when you are hot and warm you when cold; it works hard to keep out – and limit the damage caused by – ultraviolet radiation and invading microorganisms. You may not be conscious of it for much of the day, but your skin is vital to your well-being.

08:00 Rise and shine

You wake up feeling too hot. In response, the tiny blood vessels close to the surface of your skin have dilated in order to lower your internal temperature. As you head for the shower, nerve endings in your soles sense pressure and the coolness of the wooden bedroom floor. You end your shower with a quick blast of cold water and the little blood vessels in your skin constrict to prevent you from becoming too cold. You apply underarm antiperspirant deodorant: the antiperspirant temporarily stops the production of sweat, while the deodorant ensures that any sweat is odourless by inhibiting the action of bacteria on the skin.

10:30 Saturday morning shopping

After dropping the children off at their friends' house, you head for the shops. You noticed this morning that your shampoo and conditioner are running low and your facial skin seems drier than normal. The pharmacist recommends a change to your normal moisturiser. You are also concerned that you have picked up a verruca on one of your regular swimming sessions and ask the pharmacist for an over-the-counter preparation to deal with it.

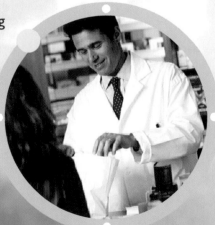

13:00 Out of the midday sun

You have a date for lunch with a friend – a regular weekend treat. But the sun is high and the day is warm, so you choose a pavement table under the awning: ultraviolet intensity is at its greatest when the sun is overhead, so you take care to stay out of the sun as much as possible between 11am and 3pm. At the very least, ultraviolet radiation hastens the development of wrinkles, which come into being when the dermis loses its elastic recoil so it doesn't snap back into shape properly. When skin is exposed to ultraviolet radiation for long periods of time on a regular basis, the elastic fibres within the dermis clump together and lose their shape.

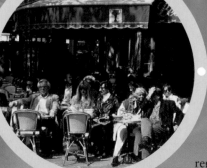

15:00 Park and ride

It's a beautiful afternoon so instead of going straight home when you pick up the kids, you all go to the park. First you make sure everyone has sunblock on any exposed skin and you slap on sunhats too. Although the peak sun hours have passed, it's still hot and after the kids have run around for half an hour, you are worried they might be overheating. Children get hot faster than adults and produce more internal heat, but their real problem is the immaturity of their sweating ability: they can't sweat enough to dissipate excess heat by evaporation. You all sit in the shade of a tree and drink a rehydrating carton of juice.

20:00 Food for friends

Back at home, you bath the children, taking care to dry them well and put them to bed. Then it's time to relax with friends over supper. For starters, you have a small portion of chicken liver pate, rich in vitamin A, a vital nutrient in preserving healthy skin. You follow this with mackerel salad – its essential fatty acids are good news for your skin. A glass of wine brings a flush to your cheeks, so you alternate with plain water, which will keep your skin and you hydrated.

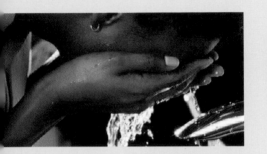 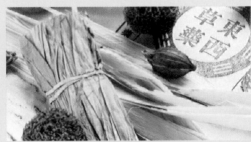 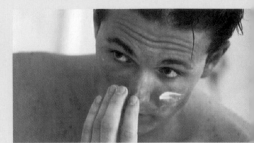

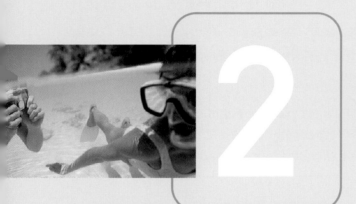

Keeping your skin, hair and nails healthy

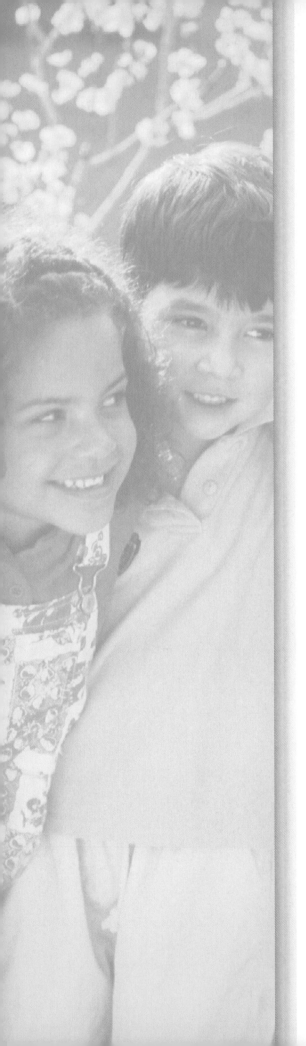

TAKE CHARGE OF YOUR SKIN HEALTH

No part of your body tells your life story better than your skin. Changes as you age, as well as many ongoing factors – work, the environment, diet, whether you smoke or drink alcohol – all affect what your skin looks and feels like. The appearance of your skin also reflects your general health.

 41 *As we get older our skin and hair change. By responding to these changes, we can keep our skin and hair in optimum condition.*

 46 *Understanding the potential damage the environment can do to skin and hair enables us to take preventative measures.*

 51 *Some medications can cause skin reactions. If starting treatment, look out for skin changes; however, most reactions soon disappear.*

 52 *Simple daily care routines can make a big difference to your skin and hair. It is not essential to use large amounts of products.*

 61 *Body hair removal can irritate the skin. Read about the methods available and recommended for different skin types and areas of the body.*

 63 *Regular nail maintenance can help to reduce the effects of environmental damage and physical stress on your nails.*

The changing face of skin and hair

Our skin and hair change as we age, due to the hormonal changes we go through and the environmental factors we are exposed to. Most of us will suffer some kind of problem with our skin and hair at some time in our lives.

HOW SKIN CHANGES WITH AGE

Some changes to the skin are intrinsic to the ageing process of the tissue itself, some are caused by influences such as hormones and disease processes, and some are due to environmental factors. In areas of the skin exposed to the environment, it is that which accounts for up to 90 per cent of the features of ageing, mainly ultraviolet radiation (UVR) from the sun.

Babies

The surface area of the skin of a newborn baby is much larger in proportion to the volume of the body, so babies are more vulnerable to heat and fluid loss than older children and adults. The skin's barrier system is not fully activated, so babies lose extra water even though their sweat glands are not yet activated.

During the first few weeks the mother's hormones are circulating and stimulate the baby's sebaceous glands. Babies also have a blood vessel system that is much more reactive so a baby's skin colour may change from pink to bright red within a few minutes. Don't overdress a baby: in hot weather a vest and nappy may be all that are needed, but watch for signs of cooling – babies cool down as fast as they overheat.

These factors mean that drugs applied to a baby's skin can be absorbed much more quickly and in larger amounts, leading to potential toxicity problems. Babies' skin is more vulnerable to chemical, physical and microbial attack because their defence systems have not matured completely.

They are prone to nappy rash, where the skin is irritated by prolonged contact with the chemicals in urine. To prevent this:
• use an effective barrier cream;
• change soiled nappies promptly;
• allow babies nappy free time to get air to their skin.

Young children

Genetic predisposition, influenced by the environment, contributes to the development of several of the most common skin diseases of childhood, such as atopic eczema. In families with a tendency to atopic problems (such as eczema, asthma and hayfever) we do not know precisely what sparks off the conditions in each individual, but these conditions are becoming much more common. Atopic eczema may be provoked by allergens such as the house dust mite or cow's milk in the diet. It was thought that avoiding cow's milk and breastfeeding a baby may reduce that risk but recent evidence may disprove this.

Less is more
When cleansing infants' skin use specially formulated products which are fragrance free and have as few ingredients as possible.

At school

As a child grows and starts nursery school, contact with infectious diseases such as chickenpox is increased. A child with chickenpox may not feel very ill, but the spots are itchy and it's very difficult for a child not to scratch. For a young child, cotton gloves may be the answer, but for an older child a cooling lotion such as calamine or aloe vera, or a cool bath can help to ease the itching.

Many activities put the skin in contact with potential irritant chemicals, and contact dermatitis can appear. Nickel allergy and rubber footwear sensitivity are examples of this type of problem. Trauma to the skin in the form of scrapes, cuts and bruises become an everyday event, but these should not be a problem if cuts are kept clean and treated with antiseptic cream.

Puberty

At puberty most teenagers suffer from spots of some sort (see below). It is important to keep the skin clean by washing gently twice a day with a mild soap. Avoid squeezing spots as this can introduce infection. Instead, apply tea tree oil to the area using a cotton bud, to gently dry spots out.

When girls gain fat during puberty, the skin on the buttocks and thighs can develop a dimpled appearance. This is known as cellulite and is completely normal for women. Although losing weight can make the dimples appear less prominent, no amount of massaging or scrubbing techniques will make any difference.

The twenties

In the twenties, skin starts to settle down after the upheaval of the teenage years, although oil (sebum) production may still be relatively high. Visible signs of ageing can start to appear towards the end of the twenties as the regenerative processes begin to slow. Skin may show a shift towards dryness and some people may notice the first lines forming around the eyes.

During the twenties a number of lifestyle choices can help to slow the effects of ageing. The most important is to reduce sun damage: limit the time spent in the sun, wear sunscreen and keep your body well-hydrated by drinking at least 2.5 litres of water a day. If you smoke, try to stop as smoking prematurely ages the skin. This is also a good time to start a skin care routine, with daily cleansing and light moisturising.

Thirty-something

During your 30s you will begin to see the first real signs of ageing as collagen and elastin fibres decrease.

Fine, dry lines show round the eyes, where the skin is at its thinnest. Increased water loss leads to drying and this decreases the skin's natural protective barrier. Broken veins show up as tiny red dots and 'smile lines' will run deeper on the side you sleep on. Lifestyle changes are less dramatic, but stress can be a critical issue. Regular late nights enjoyed in the twenties now bring puffy dark circles under the eyes.

Both men and women should wear a sunscreen of at least SPF 15, and moisturiser can be used daily. Eye creams and gels can also become useful at this stage.

The middle years

If you have taken reasonably good care of your skin, avoided excess sun and are healthy, the signs of ageing should be minor for both men and women. However, deeper lines form around the mouth and eyes, furrows appear on the forehead and age spots may develop. After the age of 45 a thinning of the skin begins. The skin looks less plump and smooth, and loses its youthful glow due to fewer blood vessels in the skin.

At this age all skincare products used should be hydrating. A rich moisturiser can help to reinvigorate tired, slack skin and improve texture.

Sixty plus

The changes in skin tone experienced in the fifties continue throughout the sixties and beyond. The skin gets drier and looser as less oil is produced, and as a result becomes more wrinkled. The skin lightens in colour due to decreased circulation and wound healing is slower. Most over-60s find that moisturiser is the best form of skin care.

10-20 YEARS

Teenagers and acne, spots and blackheads

Acne is one of the most common skin disorders, characterised by blackheads, whiteheads and pimples, especially on the face, back and chest. Acne is mainly seen in adolescents and tends to be slightly more severe in males.

Most acne is caused by an overproduction of sebum by the sebaceous glands in the skin. This is triggered by increased levels of androgen (male) hormones in both males and females during puberty.

Excess sebum can cause the follicle openings on the skin to become blocked. The sebum can harden and darken, forming blackheads. If the follicles are sealed by keratin (dead skin cells) the sebum hardens under the skin to form whiteheads. In both cases, bacteria can multiply in the sebum, causing inflammation. This attracts white blood cells that form pus; if pustules develop deep into the skin, painful nodules form.

Acne products can help by killing the bacteria that cause inflammation; if these do not work, a doctor may prescribe medication (see page 113). As acne can affect the way people feel about themselves, it is worth seeking professional help.

PREGNANCY

The hormonal changes in pregnancy can lead to a number of changes to the skin, hair and nails. Most of these are advantageous for women, although there can be downsides.

Some of the skin changes are related to the increase in blood supply to the skin. This can result in the characteristic 'glow' of pregnancy when many women say their skin feels healthier. Many women experience fewer spots and blemishes as hormonal changes can reduce sebum production. Eating better and avoiding smoking and alcohol may also pay dividends for the skin.

Skin diseases such as eczema and psoriasis may improve in pregnancy, but they can become worse. Some women find that red palms and small spider-like blood vessels can develop.

Pregnancy also brings an increase in skin pigmentation, particularly in brunettes. Areas of the skin that are already dark – such as the nipples, areolae, genital area and the midline of the abdominal wall – can become darker. Up to 70 per cent of women develop a condition called chloasma, in which the skin colour of the forehead, temples and central part of the face darkens. These changes are caused by the increase in oestrogen in the bloodstream, and usually settle down when the pregnancy ends, though some women are left with permanent changes. Mole size and activity may also increase.

Nails grow faster and can become brittle and raised from the nail bed. Massaging baby oil into the cuticles may help.

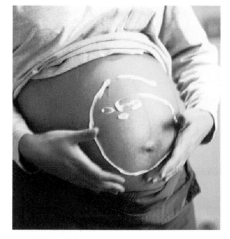

Keeping the skin supple
Some women develop stretchmarks which fade after the pregnancy but do not entirely disappear. Many women claim certain creams and lotions are effective if massaged into the skin during pregnancy, but generally whether a woman develops stretchmarks is a matter of luck: there is no really effective treatment.

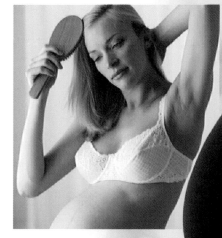

Changes to hair texture
Many women find their hair becomes thicker during pregnancy. This is because oestrogen keeps a larger proportion of hairs in the actively growing phase. Oil production increases so hair that was dry before pregnancy may become shiny; hair that was oily, however, may appear lank.

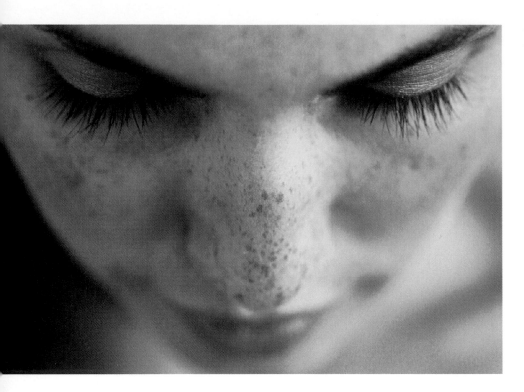

common in children, and in people with pale skin and fair or red hair. They may fade away almost completely in the winter and darken again in the sun.

Some freckles persist even in the absence of the sun; these are called lentigos, or liver spots (page 148). Despite the name, these are not linked to liver function. They tend to appear on sun-exposed sites. Liver spots usually appear during middle age – no treatment is needed but they can, rarely, be associated with the development of melanoma.

HAIR GROWTH

The rate of hair growth varies around the body. Human vellus hair grows 0.03mm in 24 hours on the male forehead, 0.21mm every 24 hours on the female thigh, 0.38mm in 24 hours on the chin of a young male, and 0.5mm per 24 hours on the crown of the scalp. Scalp hair grows faster in women than men, but faster in boys than girls before puberty. Hair may grow faster depending on age, genetics and hormonal state. Growth of body hair peaks between the ages of 50 and 69.

Straight or curly?

Whether a hair is straight or curly depends on the shape of the hair shaft. Straight hair has a circular cross-section, curly hair has a flattened elliptical cross-section, while wavy hair has a shape somewhere between a circle and a flattened ellipse. These factors vary according to racial origin.

Thinning and balding hair

As many adults age, their hair can become thinner and they experience some hair loss (see pages 85–87).

The freckle gene
Freckles are inherited and as a person ages their freckles tend to become less noticeable. Apart from sun protection, no treatment is necessary.

NORMAL FRECKLES AND MOLES

Freckles and moles are very common, and are usually harmless, pigmented spots on the skin. Birthmarks are pigmented areas of skin varying in size and colour (see page 137). The major problem for medical and lay people is deciding whether a mole may be a form of skin cancer: 30 per cent of malignant melanomas – the least common but potentially fatal form of skin cancer – arise in a pre-existing mole.

What is a mole?

Moles are collections of pigment-forming cells (melanocytes) situated in the epidermis and/ or dermis. They can be present from birth (congenital) or develop afterwards (acquired). The majority appear after birth but before the age of 20. They continue to develop and change until about the age of 40. Initially the cells are at the basal layer of the epidermis but gradually sink into the dermis, after which they grow and become raised.

It is important to check for any changes to moles that may suggest malignancy, including border and colour irregularity, and asymmetry.

Anyone who has more than about 50 moles, or who has a family history of malignant melanoma or atypical moles, should have them checked regularly by a doctor.

What are freckles?

Freckles, also called ephelides, are pale brown flat spots of concentrated pigment. They are usually less than 3mm in diameter with an irregular edge: those that seem larger may be joined to another. Freckles are more

HAIR COLOUR

Hair colour is genetically controlled. Human hair colour is under the control of at least four different genes. Dark hair predominates in the world, and ethnic differences between hair colour are very evident.

Hair pigmentation depends entirely on the presence of melanin, a pigment produced by melanocyte cells in the hair follicle, but the colour we perceive also depends on the hair's physical condition. The range of colours produced by melanin is limited to shades of yellow, brown, red and black.

Hair colour often darkens with age, so a red-headed child may darken through brown to sandy or auburn in adulthood.

Hair colour may also change because of nutritional deficiencies, particularly copper and protein deficiency. Hair also binds to inorganic elements such as copper, and a chlorinated swimming pool can turn blonde hair green. Cobalt workers can develop blue hair and indigo handlers deep blue hair. People who work with TNT sometimes develop reddish-brown hair.

The greying of hair

Greying hair is part of the ageing process and is due to a progressive reduction in melanocyte function. This results in a gradual dilution of pigment along individual hairs from normal to white and from one hair to another: this process is called canities. When there are few, if any, remaining melanocytes in the hair follicle the hair appears white. The white colour seen in the absence of melanin is due to the reflection and refraction of light on the hair; there really is no colour at all.

By the age of 50 at least half the population have at least 50 per cent grey hair. In men, the beard and moustache go grey before the hair on the head.

Close examination of greying hair frequently reveals a small precentage of white hairs among a higher percentage of normal dark pigmented hairs.

The age at which the greying process starts is genetically determined: on average it begins between the mid-30s and mid-40s. Premature greying has been defined as onset before 20 in Caucasians and 30 in Negroid people. It is thought to have a genetic base, and is commonly associated with auto-immune disorders such as pernicious anaemia and thyroid disease. Some people have localised patches of white hairs due to the absence of melanocytes or a deficiency in follicle function.

Can hair really turn white overnight?

Hair can't turn white overnight. This is because hair is dead and the only way to change its colour is with dye. However, a condition known as diffuse alopecia areata may occur to someone with a mix of white and pigmented hairs (or 'salt and pepper' hair). This condition – caused by enormous stress or emotional upheaval – results in sudden, substantial hair loss. For unknown reasons it seems to affect mostly pigmented hairs, leaving the white hairs untouched, so it appears that the person's hair has become white 'overnight'. After an episode of alopecia areata, new hairs often grow white, but become pigmented.

IT'S NOT TRUE!

'Shaving makes your hair grow faster/curly/thicker'

Shaving will not make your hair grow thicker, faster or curlier. Hair is dead protein, so cutting it won't make any difference to how it grows.

Initially hair may feel coarser after shaving, but this is due to the feel of blunt hair ends after being cut with a razor. If shaving actually increased hair growth, it would essentially be a cure for male pattern baldness, and many more men would have shaved heads in the short term.

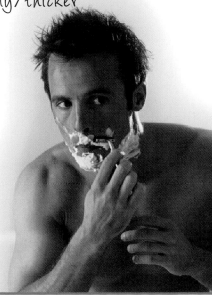

Avoiding risks to the skin and hair

Our appearance determines to a large extent how we think of ourselves, and self-image and self-esteem are vitally bound up with our looks. This makes an awareness of the factors that might harm how we look important.

A major function of the skin is to prevent the environment from damaging the body's vulnerable tissues. All parts of the skin contribute to this protective role. The skin can react in several different ways to internal illnesses and the world around us.

Many people take their skin for granted, but it has several basic needs. First, it needs to be kept clean. Second, it needs to be protected from sunlight and the environment. It shows its reaction to environmental factors in several different ways, including eczema, blistering, acne, rashes and discoloration.

Skin comes into contact with a variety of chemical substances, some of which are fairly harmless and others dangerous. And although toxic substances are capable of injuring all who come into contact with them, some individuals have more sensitive skin than others.

In general people with darker skins are less at risk from irritant damage and UV damage – fair-skinned and red-haired individuals suffer much more. The reason for these differences is not known, but people with fair skin have high UV sensitivity and are at an increased risk of developing skin problems caused by chemical irritants.

Even everyday things in places we would regard as natural and harmless can unexpectedly cause a severe problem.

HOUSEHOLD IRRITANTS

Most everyday substances such as washing-up liquid, bleach, oven cleaner and detergents are fairly harmless with occasional contact, but repeated exposure can damage the skin. These substances can penetrate and irritate the epidermis, causing dermatitis. Repeated insult leads to so-called chemical irritant eczema. This is an inflammatory response by the skin to the injury. Toxic chemicals such as acids can remove the surface layer of the skin by destroying the cells, leaving a weeping bare area or skin ulcer.

As well as eczema, chemicals may cause blistering or abnormalities in pigmentation. Depigmentation can be caused by materials that damage the pigment-producing cells, such as some rubber additives.

People with sensitive skin find that some cosmetic products cause irritant or allergic reactions. The preparations most likely to cause a problem are eye and facial cosmetics, deodorants, hair dyes and soaps. If a reaction occurs, cosmetics should not be used and, if necessary, topical steroid cream will be prescribed until the reaction subsides.

DOMESTIC IRRITATIONS

At home or in the garden the skin can be exposed to many irritant substances. Regular assault can damage the skin's protective barriers, so it is always best to take preventative measures.

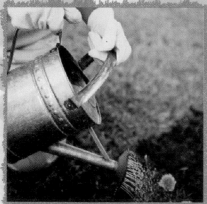

COVER UP
While gardening wear protective gloves to protect the skin from scratches and contact with any chemicals.

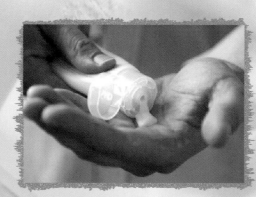

BE KIND TO YOUR HANDS
Rubbing in moisturiser will help to rehydrate the skin, and it can also provide an effective barrier to prevent further moisture loss.

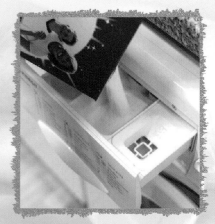

BE LAUNDRY WISE
If you have sensitive skin use non-biological powder and double rinse your clothes, to remove residue.

What you can do

- Avoid prolonged exposure to potential irritants: wear gloves when handling chemicals.
- Wash and dry hands thoroughly and use a moisturiser; massage it well into the nails and cuticles too.
- If you have sensitive skin use hypoallergenic products (page 54).

GARDEN HAZARDS

Our lives are inextricably bound up with plants, whether we are growing them, cooking and eating them, or arranging them for display. Some occupations bring people into daily contact with potentially hazardous plants and woods. People at risk from occupational skin problems include gardeners, nursery workers, fruit pickers, florists, flower arrangers, greengrocers, farmers, foresters and botanists.

Some plants are known to cause skin rashes and it may be that they have survived better for being dangerous to pick or eat. More commonly, however, the reaction may be caused by a chemical the plant produces. Plants that are known to cause irritant eczema include primulas, ivy, Euphorbia, daffodil bulbs, and Dieffenbachia, a common office plant. Other plants only cause problems when we are also in the sun. Such phototoxic reactions are caused by a relatively small number of species, including:

- **Umbelliferae** Vegetables such as celery, carrot and parsnip, herbs such as dill, cumin and parsley, ornamental plants and weeds such as cow parsley and giant hogweed.
- **Rutaceae** These include citrus fruits, rue and burning bush.
- **Figs**

The chemical involved in all these reactions is psoralens, a natural fungicide produced by plants. This interacts with the DNA of mammalian cells and when UVR falls on the area it can produce an acute inflamed blistered area of skin. The skin rash urticaria can be produced by some plants such as the stinging nettle injecting the irritant into the skin; the rash appears at the point of contact. In other cases eating the plant can provoke urticaria all over the body. Foods such as green peppers, strawberries, onions and tomatoes may cause such reactions.

Skin reactions when gardening can also be caused by such irritants as rubber in gloves, or the stinging hairs of the brown-tail moth which lives quietly in garden sheds.

Weedkillers and insecticides can damage the nails. This can vary from causing a white band across the nail to total loss of the nail.

What you can do

- Wear non-latex gloves when you are gardening.
- Avoid foods which cause a rash.
- Avoid the sun when gardening: choose cool, dull times of day.
- Use organic weedkillers and check the safety of any insecticides used.
- Don't grow those plants that cause skin irritation: if they are already in your garden, have someone remove them.

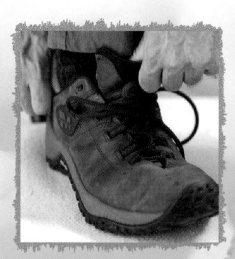

CHOOSE SHOES WITH CARE
To keep the skin on your feet healthy, buy shoes made from breathable materials such as leather or canvas.

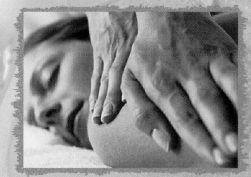

TAKE TIME OUT
Massage is a soothing form of relaxation, while the firm but gentle hand movements increase oxygen and blood flow to the skin.

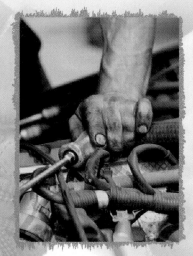

OIL CLEAN-UP
Lubricating oils used by mechanics can cause acne and dermatitis, so clean the skin thoroughly.

- Expect sizes to vary according to style and construction – don't assume you always wear the same size, choose the size that fits best.
- Check that you can wiggle your toes when wearing the shoes.

Calluses can also affect the hands, and may develop to protect the underlying tissues.

Forgotten feet

If you spend all day on your feet, fill a large bowl with warm water and add some bubble bath for a soothing and relaxing foot spa.

SHOES AND THE SKIN

Many minor but painful foot problems such as calluses and corns are caused by poorly fitting shoes. These small pads of hard skin develop at sites under pressure. People who spend their time walking barefoot are prone to developing large areas of thickened skin on the soles of the feet. These develop as a way for the foot to protect itself from injury, but can become cracked, painful and infected.

When buying shoes:
- Choose leather or canvas: both materials breathe and mould to your feet.
- Always have your feet measured; feet can spread with age so your shoe size may alter over the years.
- Shop for shoes at the end of the day, when your feet will have swollen to their maximum extent.

STRESS AND THE SKIN

It is generally believed that stress can cause illness, and this applies to skin conditions too. Stress can exacerbate several pre-existing skin conditions such as acne, psoriasis and rosacea. It is also believed that outbreaks of these conditions can be triggered by a single stressful event.

There is also a self-induced skin disease, dermatitis artefacta, which may be related to psychological problems. Picking, scratching and rubbing the skin, pulling out hair and damaging nails by picking can all lead to serious skin problems.

One of the best things you can do for the health of your body, which will also have a positive impact on your skin, is to find out what stresses you and take steps to relieve it.

Relief strategies
- Take a break.
- Buy a self-help book or video.
- Learn to meditate or do yoga.
- Eat well and avoid alcohol.
- Get enough sleep.

YOUR OCCUPATION AND YOUR SKIN

An occupational skin disease (OSD) is any skin disorder which is caused by a person's work. A person's existing skin disorder may also be made worse by work activities and such cases are also considered to be OSDs. Skin diseases are one of the most common forms of work-induced illness, so it is important to know whether you are at risk from the type of work that you do.

Skin reactions account for 40 per cent of all occupational diseases.

Examples of occupational skin problems include:
- contact dermatitis;
- irritant and allergic dermatitis;
- worsening of pre-existing skin diseases such as eczema.

Some skin cancers are also related to occupations. In the UK it has been estimated that 4 million working days are lost each year due to employees taking time off work because of skin disorders.

Occupations with the highest risk include hairdressers, printers, nurses, foundry workers, beauticians, machine tool operators, chemical and biological scientists, electroplaters and vehicle assemblers. Anyone who has a past history of eczema as a child might be advised to think carefully before pursuing these occupations.

Nails can also be damaged in occupations such as hairdressing, while artificial nail appliers have been known to develop sensitivity to the adhesive.

OBESITY

The skin is affected by obesity. Conditions such as intertrigo – skin infections of the groin, under the breasts, in the armpits – are common, as microorganisms can flourish in the warm, moist areas created by folds of fat.

People who are seriously overweight can develop stretch marks in the abdomen and thighs, which resemble those that occur in pregnancy. They are particularly common in adolescents who gain weight quickly and usually become less obvious after weight is lost.

People with severe obesity may develop insulin resistance, thought to be the precursor to type II diabetes. Various skin problems are associated with this, including a thickening and darkening of skin creases.

Irritating work
Hairdressers come into contact with a wide range of chemicals which can damage the surface layer of the skin and cause eczema.

SMOKING

Collagen fibres form the structural support in the dermis of the skin and are constantly being renewed. Smoking impedes this process, leading to premature ageing of the skin's appearance. Smoking also reduces the blood supply to the skin by damaging the frail membrane lining the arteries. This can lead to loss of skin hair on the legs, shiny fragile skin and delayed healing. The toenails can become thickened and deformed, and fingernails can split. The arch of the foot may also distort, leading to ulcers on the toes. This is many times worse in someone who already has diabetes.

A yellowish hair colour is not uncommon in white or grey-haired heavy smokers due to the tar in cigarette smoke. The fingernails and fingers can be heavily discoloured yellow and brown, stained by the tar.

The best advice for your skin is not to smoke, or if you do, to use every available resource to stop.

ALCOHOL

Alcohol has the reputation of giving people a red face. In fact alcohol, hot drinks, spicy foods, emotion, UV light, and extremes of temperature can all precipitate flushing in a vulnerable individual. The blood vessels of the skin dilate, bringing extra blood to the skin surface, so the skin reddens and feels warm. For most people, alcohol related flushing is only temporary and fades after a few hours.

In some people the small blood vessels become fixed in dilation, so that they appear red-faced and have tiny broken blood vessels on the skin of the face all the time. Alcohol may also raise the body's temperature, causing sweating.

Heavy drinking can lead to a dry, dull complexion. This is due to the dehydrating effects of alcohol, and is more noticeable in women. Minor skin infections are also more common because alcohol weakens the body's natural defence system. Alcohol poisoning is indicated by cold, clammy, pale or bluish skin.

It is important to drink only in moderation (no more than two drinks a day for a woman, and three for a man, and always have one or two alcohol-free days each week).

STREET DRUGS

Street drugs can cause severe damage to the skin. Inhaling solvents such as glue can permanently injure the delicate lining of the nasal cavity, and cause sores to form around the nose and mouth. These sores may be the first clue that someone is trying these substances.

Injecting drugs with non-sterile needles can give rise to bacterial skin infections, abscesses and cellulitis.

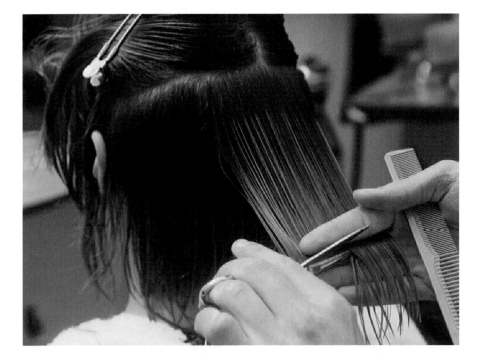

EXERCISE AND HOBBIES

Although exercise is obviously good for general health it can generate a few problems as far as the skin and nails are concerned. Awareness of potential problems is the first step to avoiding them. In almost all cases a few simple precautions are all you need to make sure that your exercise is not causing problems for your skin and nails.

Jogger's nipple
Petroleum jelly applied to the nipples before a run may prevent jogger's nipple, an eczema-like condition caused by friction from clothing allied with increased sweat levels. For women a correctly fitting sports bra may help.

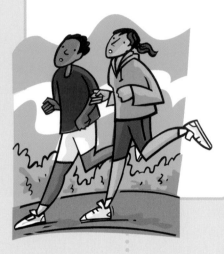

Calluses and corns
For any sport, including walking, get good advice on the correct footwear from an experienced person, and be sure that shoes fit well. Badly fitting sports shoes can cause the formation of hard pads of skin which need careful treatment by a chiropodist.

Musician's neck
Fiddler's neck is a well-recognised skin problem found in professional violin and viola players. Friction from the chin rest can lead to a form of eczema, and an acne-like cyst. In some cases, acne medication can be used to treat the condition; the cyst can be surgically removed.

Toenail dystrophy
It is important to be aware that when we run, walk fast or dance our feet go forward into the front of our shoes. This can lead to recurrent impact of the toe into the shoe, causing damage to the nail bed, where the nail is formed. The toenail can be severely thickened and misshapen. Prevention is better than cure, so ensuring shoes fit well is a good first step. Anyone who is doing heavy manual work should wear shoes with steel toecaps.

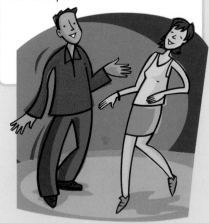

Athlete's foot
Exercise causes increased perspiration, and this encourages the growth of fungus between the toes, giving rise to the condition known as athlete's foot. This can be prevented by wearing cotton socks and scrupulously drying the feet after exercise. OTC powders help to ensure the feet are completely dry and creams eradicate the fungus.

Medication and the skin

Almost any drug can cause a skin reaction, and many inflammatory skin diseases can be caused or made worse by drugs. Knowing about possible reactions can help you and your doctor to pinpoint the likely culprit.

Some, but not all, drug reactions are due to allergy. Others are due to overdose or to the accumulation of a drug in the skin. Some are unwanted side effects of an otherwise useful drug. Some drugs are much more likely to cause skin reactions as a side effect than others. Ask your doctor or pharmacist about possible side effects for your skin before taking any new drug: if you suddenly develop a skin problem soon after starting a new drug, check with your pharmacist whether it could be to blame and seek your doctor's advice on whether to continue taking it.

There are a number of well-defined skin reaction patterns associated with specific drugs.

RED ITCHY RASHES
The most common skin reactions to drugs are itchy, widespread, red bumpy rashes. In most cases the rash erupts after a few days on the drug, but sometimes there is a delay of a few weeks. Stopping the drug usually leads to the subsiding of the rash within a week. Drugs that commonly cause this rash include the antibiotic amoxycillin and NSAIDs.

URTICARIA AND ANAPHYLAXIS
Occasionally drugs may produce a severe allergic reaction within minutes of taking them, and this can be very serious. If you have had such a reaction in the past, you must carry an adrenaline injection for self-administration (an Epipen, available

on prescription) and an alerting bracelet or other notification. Drugs that may cause this reaction include aspirin, penicillin, morphine and codeine.

ECZEMA
Contact dermatitis can be caused by the ingredients of topical creams and ointments. Lanolin, preservatives such as parabens, topical anaesthetics, antihistamines and antibiotics can all cause this reaction.

PHOTOTOXICITY
Some drugs increase the skin's sensitivity to the sun, so it can burn even on an overcast day. Examples of this are tetracycline antibiotics, oral contraceptives, and the thiazide drugs used for high blood pressure.

Drugs, topical or taken internally, and chemicals on the skin can interact with UVR and cause

immunological reactions – usually contact eczema. The eruption will only occur on areas of the body exposed to light such as the backs of the hands, the neck, nose, chin and the forehead. This usually occurs after the second or third exposure to UVR, and is often delayed by 2–3 weeks, so it can be difficult to work out the cause of these sorts of rashes.

HAIR LOSS
This commonly happens when people are given cytotoxic drugs to treat cancer. Hair nearly always regrows after treatment is finished. Some drugs such as warfarin, anti-thyroid drugs and the contraceptive pill can cause hair thinning.

SKIN PIGMENTATION CHANGES
Increased skin pigmentation may happen with photosensitivity, but some commonly used drugs can cause other types of pigment to be deposited in the skin. Minocycline, used to treat acne, may leave reversible blue deposits on scarred areas such as the face or shins.

SAFETY WITH HERBAL MEDICATIONS
Chinese herbs have proven successful in treating eczema and psoriasis in children. If you are going to try this treatment, doctors recommend buying the herbs from a reputable practitoner who uses only 'standardised ingredients'. If the ingredients are not standardised you have no way of gauging how your body will react to them. Once a course of treatment is started, doctors recommend regular blood tests to monitor liver function.

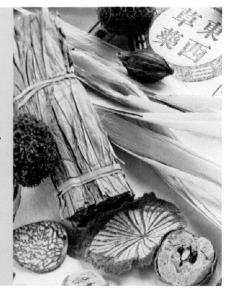

Skin and hair care basics

Eating a balanced diet, drinking plenty of water, avoiding smoking and excess alcohol, exercising regularly and getting enough sleep – all these contribute to healthy skin, especially when backed up by an effective skin care routine.

Effective skin care should cleanse the skin regularly and replenish the moisture in its uppermost layers.

There are many skin care products on the market and choosing what suits you can be a daunting prospect. You need to have a good idea what you are looking for before you start.

Skin care should also include protecting your skin against the harmful effects of ultraviolet (UV) rays by applying products that offer UV protection (see page 76).

Facial skincare for men
In the not too distant past the concept of skin products especially for men seemed unthinkable. Today, ranges for men include cleansers, moisturisers and astringents. The male skin needs at least as much care as female skin, perhaps more. Male skin is more prone to excessive oil production, and the regular use of deep-skin cleansers can help to keep the skin in optimum condition.

SKIN TYPES
Sebaceous skin glands – especially those on the forehead, and around the eyes, nose and chin – produce sebum, a natural oil; the amount that is produced determines your skin type. If sebum fills the gaps between the dead surface cells, this results in a normal texture skin. If less oil is produced the skin feels rougher; this is dry skin. If the glands are extra active the skin is oily, but if this oil is only on the forehead, nose and chin, this is called combination skin. Different skin types need different skin care routines (see panel below).

SOAPS AND FACE WASHES
Normal soaps contain detergents that are harsh on the skin and reduce the amount of water and natural oils in its uppermost layers. This means that using soap and water on the face may leave the skin feeling tight and dry, particularly if you tend to have dry skin anyway. Alternative soaps and face washes are available that cleanse the skin without the use of detergents and contain moisturisers. For oily and spotty skin, medicated soaps and washes containing specially formulated gentle detergents can be beneficial.

DAILY CARE FOR THE FACE

Although skin care regimes differ according to skin type, there are two basic steps that should be carried out by everyone. First, cleansing the skin of makeup, and second, moisturising to help to keep the skin supple and prevent moisture loss. Toning is not an essential part of skin care but many people choose to use a toner to clear any residual makeup and freshen the skin before moisturiser is applied. In addition, exfoliation is considered a valuable measure for achieving healthy, glowing skin. Skin type can change through life and a skin care routine may need to be modified accordingly. For example, oily skin may develop at certain times in life, particularly during the teenage years, but may not be permanent – skin generally becomes drier with age.

Normal skin
If you are one of those fortunate people who have normal skin, you still need to follow a daily skin care regime to ensure that it stays that way. The skin should be thoroughly cleansed twice a day. Cleansers that are washed away with water are suitable and leave the skin feeling refreshed. Toners with alcohol should be avoided for normal skin; alcohol can dry the skin and leave it feeling tight and uncomfortable. Oil-in-water moisturising creams or lotions are perfect for normal skin, and are light and easily applied. The face can be exfoliated once a week to clear some of the dead cells on the surface. A mask can also be applied once a week. Various types of skin masks are available for normal skin and can be used in turn for a hydrating boost (a moisturising mask) or for deeper cleansing (a clay mask).

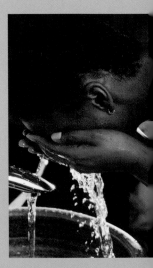

SKIN CLEANSERS

Skin cleansers gently remove makeup and daily grime from the face without the use of detergents. They can be used in place of soaps and are available in a number of forms, including creams and lotions that are applied to the skin and wiped off with cotton wool pads. Foaming washes are washed away with water, leaving the skin feeling refreshed. However, some people with dry skin find that even water can leave their face feeling tight and uncomfortable. If you are one of those people, you may find cleansing creams and lotions preferable.

TONER

A toner removes any remaining cleansing residue, closes pores and returns the skin to its proper pH balance. The skin is then smooth and ready to absorb a moisturiser.

FACIAL SCRUBS

The small, smooth granules in facial scrubs remove the dead cells from the skin surface (exfoliation), helping moisture to enter and giving the skin a healthy glow. The scrub is rubbed over the face with gentle circular movements, avoiding the skin in the delicate eye area. This should be done no more than once a week.

The whole body can benefit from exfoliation. Body scrubs usually contain larger, slightly rougher granules than those found in facial scrubs. The body can be exfoliated two to three times a week.

FACE PACKS

These provide an intensive treatment, whether your skin needs a moisture boost or deep cleansing, or a combination of the two. Masks are available in various forms, including thick creams and formulations designed to harden, then peel off. Leaving the mask on for a period of time means that the skin derives maximum benefit from the ingredients. Special eye masks are available to treat the delicate skin around the eyes. A weekly face pack treatment can benefit most skins.

MOISTURISERS

Applying moisturiser regularly is a vital part of skin care. These products are available in many different forms, and some are more effective than others.

What does a moisturiser do?

Moisturisers replenish the moisture and oils in the upper layers of the skin and provide a protective layer on the skin's surface to prevent moisture loss. Some moisturisers give protection against ultraviolet rays, reducing their damaging and ageing

---

Oily skin

The skin should be cleansed twice a day with a face wash containing gentle detergents. If a toner is used, use one specially formulated for oily skin which can slightly reduce the natural oils (sebum), which are present in excess in oily skin. Even oily skin needs to be moisturised regularly. Water-soluble moisturisers that are light and easy to apply are usually preferable. The skin can be exfoliated and a deep cleansing clay mask applied once a week.

Dry skin

Dry skin products should contain ingredients that add and retain water in the skin's upper layers. Use a mild cleanser that contains no detergents and if a toner is used it should not contain alcohol. If the face is washed, the water should be warm, never hot. Moisturise twice daily with an intensive moisturiser.

Combination skin

Cleansers are available that are suited to combination skin. Cleansing can be followed by a mild toner applied to the oily areas. The whole of the face, including the oily parts, then needs to be moisturised. An oil-inhibiting moisturiser will hydrate the dry cheeks adequately without making the oily central panel of the face more greasy. Extra moisture may sometimes be needed by the dry areas of the face. This can be achieved by applying a more intensive moisturiser rich in humectants. The face can be exfoliated gently once a week. Masks are available that are specially formulated to suit both dry and greasy skin. Alternatively, two masks may be used: clay for the oily areas and a moisturising mask for dry patches.

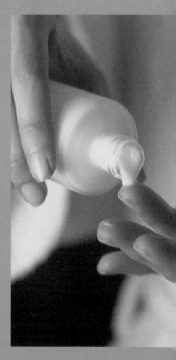

As aloe vera gel is 90 per cent water it is excellent for soothing and rehydrating the skin. Other ingredients include minerals, vitamins, enzymes and amino acids.

effect on the skin. Everyone – but particularly people over the age of 30 years and those with dry skin – should use a moisturiser with SPF 20 or higher every day.

A good moisturiser will make the skin feel softer and should relieve dryness without making the skin feel greasy. If you tend to have dry skin, the 'tight' feeling should be relieved.

The skin of the face should be moisturised twice a day: in the morning to replenish moisture after washing or cleansing, and especially at the end of the day when the face should be fully cleansed and a moisturiser applied.

Ideally, the body should be moisturised daily after a shower or bath when the skin is still damp. Moisturising the body twice a day is beneficial, particularly for those who have dry skin.

Which type shall I use?

There are so many moisturisers available, it can be difficult to know which to choose, but you need to bear two things in mind: first, your skin type, and second, how much time you have available to care for it.

Creams tend to be the more intensive form of treatment. They are usually thick and for this reason may take a little longer to apply than more liquid preparations. Creams are often oil-based and are particularly suitable for skins that tend to be dry.

For normal and combination skins, lotions should provide adequate moisture. Lotions are light, easy to apply and dry quickly. Some people with combination skin like to apply more intensive cream to the drier areas of the face, such as the cheeks, although combination skin products are made to suit all areas.

Gels are usually water-based and are particularly helpful for greasy or sensitive skin. They are light and easy to use, and do not add extra oil which could overload the skin.

In addition, some moisturisers are available in two forms: day and night creams. For young people it may be enough to use the same cream or lotion morning and night. Those over the age of 30 years and people with dry skin, may find it beneficial to use a thicker, more intensive treatment before bed.

HYPOALLERGENIC PRODUCTS

If you have sensitive skin, it is worth buying hypoallergenic products. These are made from highly purified ingredients and do not contain well-known allergens – ingredients that are known to be capable of causing

allergic reactions. However, 'hypo' means less, not none: hypoallergenic products contain fewer potential irritants or allergens, not none at all. Some people find plant-based hypoallergenic products cause fewer reactions on sensitive skin.

ANTI-WRINKLE CREAMS

Many cosmetics companies claim that their moisturisers can halt the effects of time, and actually reduce the appearance of fine lines and wrinkles. However, many of these products do little more than act as a kind of skin 'Polyfilla', smoothing out the wrinkles by filling in the cracks between them. Other products contain AHAs (alpha-hydroxy acids), plant-derived ingredients that help to remove dead skin cells from the skin surface. As far as skin health is concerned, the important factor is not the appearance of lines but maintaining a sufficient moisture level in the skin.

BEFORE YOU BUY

When choosing a skin care product it is worth reading the information on the label. Not only will this tell you whether the product is suitable for your skin type, it may also give valuable additional information, such as whether it gives UV protection.

If you are buying something for the first time, try the tester if one is available, then buy the smallest size possible. If the product suits you can then invest in a larger economy size – and if it doesn't, you haven't wasted too much money.

BODY BRUSHING

Body brushing stimulates the blood circulation to the skin and improves skin tone. It is only suitable for the body as the skin of the face is too delicate. Body brushing treatment should be done in a warm room with the skin completely dry. A soft brush is swept firmly over the body, starting from the feet and working upwards. The brushing should be followed by moisturising.

CARING FOR THE HANDS

The skin on the hands tends to age rapidly as it is frequently washed, comes into contact with all manner of substances and is the skin most often exposed to damaging ultraviolet rays. In addition, the layer of natural oils protecting the back of the hand is thin, so that moisture is easily lost. This makes moisturising the hands an important part of skin care that may need to be done several times a day.

Moisturisers containing humectants such as glycerin replenish the moisture within the skin; petroleum jelly and other so-called occlusives reduce moisture loss. AHAs help to remove the outer layer of dead cells and encourage the production of new skin cells.

In addition, massaging the hands when applying moisturiser increases the blood supply to the skin and so improves its condition. The nails also need attention and regular maintenance (see pages 63–64).

FEET AND FOOT CARE

As our feet are hidden from view for most of the day, we tend to forget about them, but skin on the feet, and particularly the heels, is vulnerable to dryness and cracking. This tends to worsen as we get older. Our feet are also prone to develop patches of hard skin. This can be reduced by wearing comfortable shoes that don't squash or pinch but support the foot.

Feet benefit from being washed and moisturised with foot lotion every day. Care should be taken when drying the feet – the skin between the toes needs to be dried thoroughly. Gently rubbing the skin with a foot file or pumice stone twice a week will reduce hard skin. Foot spas can relax tired feet and improve the condition of the skin – the warm water and the massaging effect increases the flow of blood to the skin. A soak in a bowl of warm water can also relieve tired feet.

PROBLEM AREAS

The heels, elbows and knees tend to get particularly dry and need special attention to prevent painful cracking. Gentle exfoliation with a body scrub every few days, and massaging every day with a moisturising cream that is rich in humectants will help to keep the skin soft and supple. Fresh lemon juice applied with a cotton pad can also help to soften the skin – these areas should then be washed and dried carefully.

CHOOSING DEODORANTS AND ANTIPERSPIRANTS

It is down to personal preference whether you choose a spray or a roll-on product. If you are prone to dryness and skin irritation, an unperfumed, hypoallergenic product is best. Many products also have hydrating properties to relieve dry skin. If you have very sensitive skin, it may take you a while to find a product that leaves your skin feeling comfortable and soft.

SKIN CARE FOR MEN

Skin products are available that are specially formulated to suit men's skin and many men are now aware of the benefits of regular skin care.

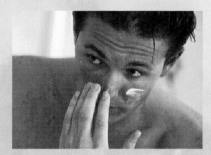

Moisturiser can help to keep the skin well-hydrated and supple. Men should consider using a moisturiser that offers UV protection, particularly when spending time outdoors.

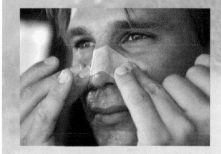

Men tend to have larger skin pores and when these become blocked with debris, spots can form. Pore cleansing strips gently peel away and remove blackheads without damaging the skin.

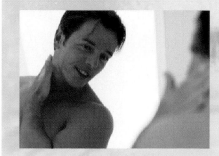

Aftershave acts as an astringent and toner for the skin. It helps to return the skin to a slightly acidic state after using alkaline shaving soaps. It also softens and smooths the skin by closing the pores.

SHAMPOOING YOUR HAIR

Hair can be washed daily without any problems provided a few simple care rules are followed. Do not use very hot water and when drying do not rub vigorously or use excessive heat. Poor-quality hair products are not good for the hair and are a false economy.

Let your hair hang naturally while you wash it. Stand in the shower or lean your head over the bath. Do not pile your hair onto the top of your head. This causes tangling and breakage.

It is best to let hair dry naturally, but if you prefer to use a dryer, use on a low setting only. Keep the dryer moving to prevent any damage to the hair shaft.

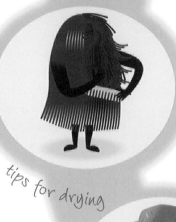

While the hair is damp, loosen tangles with a wide-toothed comb. Taking a section of hair at a time, use gentle downward strokes. Start near the ends and work towards the roots, hold the hair just above the section you are combing to prevent dragging.

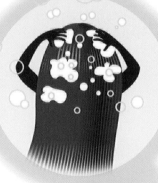

Using warm water, rinse your hair thoroughly to prepare for shampooing.

Do not apply shampoo direct to your hair from the bottle, but pour some into the palm of your hand.

tips for shampooing

tips for drying

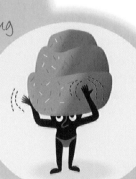

Wrap a clean towel around your hair and pat dry using a blotting action. Do not rub vigorously, this will cause tangling and breakage.

Gently rub the shampoo between your palms. Starting at the scalp, work the shampoo into your hair gently with your fingers in a claw-like shape.

Leave the conditioner on for two minutes, then rinse well.

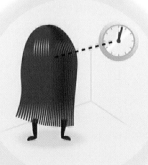

tips for conditioning

Rinse your hair well to remove all traces of shampoo, allowing the water to cascade through the hair. Do not rub your wet hair.

Pour some conditioner into the palm of your hand, spread it between the palms then work it into the hair gently, evenly and thoroughly.

HAIR CARE

Not only is there is a right way to shampoo and condition hair to keep it healthy, but different hair types respond to different treatments.

DRY, GREASY OR NORMAL?

In addition to basic type – straight, wavy or tightly curled (see page 44) – hair can be normal, dry or greasy. The quality and feel of hair changes with age, stress and trauma, and also depend on how you treat the hair.

Dry hair

Dry hair does not shine and feels rough to the touch. It tangles easily, is prone to split ends and is difficult to style. This is because it does not contain enough moisture – the outer layer of the hair (the cuticle layer) has become porous so the inside of the hair (the cortex) cannot retain water. The condition is more common in longer hair than short, since it has been growing for longer and has been subjected to greater cosmetic and environmental trauma. In addition, chemical treatments such as perming, colouring and bleaching cause dryness. Dry hair should be treated with mild shampoos and conditioners. It also responds to intensive restructuring conditioners. These usually contain panthenol, which has a cumulative effect on the hair shaft helping it to retain moisture, and proteins which help to smooth the cuticle layer.

Greasy hair

The feel of the hair depends on the amount of grease present. Greasy hair tends to be limp, looks flat and has little volume. It soon gets greasy again after shampooing, owing to a build-up of sebum produced by the sebaceous glands in the scalp. Sebum is a natural oil which passes into the hair follicle and over the hair shaft. It does not penetrate the hair shaft but lies on its surface.

The amount of sebum produced by the body fluctuates: it is more abundant during puberty, for example, when there tends to be a higher level of male hormones present. It has been suggested that stress may increase the amount of sebum produced, as can poor-quality shampoos. It is not possible to stop the glands producing sebum, nor does diet affect its production. The best course is to use a shampoo designed for greasy hair and wash hair daily, before too much grease has a chance to build up.

Normal hair

Normal hair is usually defined as hair that has not had any chemical applications and is neither greasy nor dry. The hair shines and is manageable, it looks good and healthy. To care for normal hair use a mild shampoo and, if the hair is longer than 15cm (6in), perhaps a little conditioner on the middle lengths to ends, which will help to soften environmental weathering.

SHAMPOOS AND CONDITIONERS

Shampoo produces lather which aids the removal of dirt from the hair by trapping dirt particles and stopping them being re-deposited on the hair. For a shampoo to be effective it must be able to remove grease and dirt from the hair without removing natural oils from the scalp. It must also be mild to avoid damaging the scalp, hair or eyes.

Shampoos

The various components of shampoo each have a specific job.
- **Cleansing agents** remove grease and dirt from the hair. Two of the milder cleansing agents used are ammonium lauryl sulphate and ammonium laureth sulphate.
- **Hair-care additives** might include anti-dandruff agents, moisturisers, herbal extracts and fruit extracts.
- **Functional additives** include preservatives, perfumes, colours, and pH controllers.

Conditioners

Most shampoos contain a degree of conditioning agent, and this is usually sufficient for people with shorter, normal hair. For longer hair, hair which has been affected by environmental trauma, or hair that has been subjected to chemical applications or over-drying, more conditioning may be necessary to improve feel and manageability.

IT'S NOT TRUE!

'The more I wash my hair, the more greasy it becomes'

Washing hair frequently does not cause more oil to be produced. Irregular shampooing, however, will result in a build-up of grease as environmental dirt sticks to the oily surface of the hair, so it is best to wash greasy hair daily using a shampoo designed for greasy hair. Such shampoos are formulated to remove natural grease without damaging the hair shaft.

Conditioners help to smooth the outside layer (the cuticle) of the hair and to reduce static electricity which causes 'fly-away' hair. They may also contain panthenol and silicones, which increase the moisture-holding properties of the hair, and smooth the hair shaft. This reduces tangling and makes the hair softer. Conditioner leaves hair easier to comb when wet or dry, which is immensely important for dry, permed, bleached or coloured hair.

Home treatment can also be applied using vegetable oil. Almond, corn and sunflower are all light oils which are easy to remove from the hair by shampooing. Pour 100ml (3fl oz) of oil into a suitable container and warm gently to lukewarm. Apply to the hair, massage and leave for 30 minutes. Remove the oil using a mild shampoo in the normal way. This can be done 2–3 times weekly.

Product build-up

Some hair products cause a gradual build-up of residue on the hair, making it look dull and limp. This can be avoided by regularly changing your hair products or by using an anti-residue shampoo once a week.

COMMON PROBLEMS

The two most common problems affecting hair are dandruff and head lice. Dandruff affects people at any age, irrespective of hair type. Head lice can affect anyone, but are more common among school children.

Dandruff

This is a problem caused by flaking of the top layer of skin on the scalp. This flaking occurs all over the body, all of the time: millions of tiny flakes are lost every day. The purpose of this is to remove skin bacteria, keeping the numbers on the skin to a minimum. On the scalp, the hair can trap these flakes and they build up or accumulate into larger flakes. The damp warm conditions that result are favourable to the multiplication of bacteria and yeasts, and can exacerbate the problem.

The best way to control dandruff is by using a shampoo containing piroctone olamine or zinc pirithione. Use daily and leave on the scalp for 2–3 minutes before rinsing. If the treatment is ineffective after two weeks, it is best to visit your doctor.

Do combined shampoos and conditioners work?

Combined shampoos and conditioners are extremely convenient as they save on storage space and time, and are useful products to take travelling. They are, however, not particularly effective for cleaning the hair.

When a normal shampoo is lathered on wet hair, it lifts the dirt and grime from the follicles. When the lather is rinsed, the dirt is rinsed away. It is only after the hair has been cleaned properly that it is ready to be conditioned.

Combined shampoos and conditioners might make your hair feel conditioned, but that is deceptive. The chemical producing the effect is building a waxy coating over the follicles that will eventually make them look dull. It is best not to use these products on a regular basis.

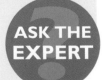

ASK THE EXPERT

HEAD LICE

There are more than 100,000 cases of head lice in the UK each year. Head lice are highly contagious and, if one person in a family becomes infected, everyone in the household must be treated.

There are five things you should know about lice and nits:
- Lice are the insects and nits are the eggs.
- It is impossible to drown lice.
- Nits are harder to eliminate than lice. This is why treatment should not be interrupted.
- Nits should not be confused with dandruff. Nits are stuck to the hair, while dandruff flakes off.
- Empty eggs are white. Live eggs are the same colour as the hair and so are harder to see.

Nearly all lice treatments are available over the counter. A single application will usually kill all head lice, taking about 12 hours to clear the problem. A second application is necessary 10 days later to kill any newly hatched nits.

Alcohol-based pesticide solutions are the most effective, but water-based alternatives are available for small children and eczema or asthma sufferers. Problems arising from overuse are only likely if manufacturer's instructions are not followed correctly.

Alternative lice treatments

For those with concerns about using pesticides on children's heads, there are alternative methods for getting rid of lice (some are shown right). They are as effective as chemical methods, but tend to be more time-consuming.

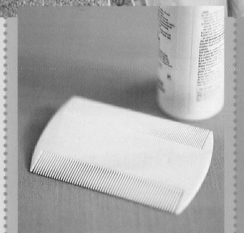

Aromatherapy oils

Many oils will kill lice, including eucalyptus, geranium, parsley, Scotch pine, rosemary, lavender, thyme and tea tree. The safest to use on children are tea tree and lavender.

In a small bottle mix 5ml (1tsp) pure tea tree or lavender essential oil, with 65ml (5tbsp) warm water, 25ml (2tbsp) pure spirit or vodka and 5ml (1tsp) castor oil. Shake the bottle well, then make a series of 1cm (½in) partings in the hair. Apply the lotion over the scalp covering approximately 5cm (2in) up the hair shaft from the roots and leave for 12 hours or overnight. Shampoo using warm water, massaging well into the scalp. Rinse and repeat. Comb through the hair with a nit comb to remove dead lice and egg cases. If possible leave hair to dry naturally, as heat will evaporate the active ingredients. Repeat every three days for two weeks and check regularly for any re-infestation. Swimming pool chlorine, perms and hair colouring can reduce the effectiveness of the treatment.

Bug Buster kit

Available from all good pharmacies, this is a special comb that is used on wet hair that has been coated with conditioner. The slippery surface makes the lice slower moving and unable to grip onto the scalp, so the comb can hook them out. Six bug-busting sessions over a two-week period should clear the problem. Unlike chemical treatments, lice cannot become resistant to bug busting.

Electronic comb

This battery-powered comb has a tiny sensor on the tip of each tooth. It can hardly be felt by humans but, as soon as the sensor touches a head louse, an electric current is released which kills it. The dead lice are caught in the teeth of the comb and are easily removed. Because the comb does not kill the eggs it is necessary to repeat the treatment every two days for two weeks. Electronic combs are difficult to use – and therefore less successful – on long hair.

CUTTING HAIR

Human hair does not grow at the same rate throughout the scalp. Some hairs will be in the middle of a growing phase, while others are coming to the end of their phase when growth is slower. This means that hair will start to look a little untidy again some 6–8 weeks after a hair cut, and it's time to revisit your hair stylist.

If you are in the process of growing your hair long, it will still need a trim every two months to tidy up the ends. In two months your hair grows an average of 2.5cm (1in). If you do not want to lose all the growth you have gained between cuts your hairdresser should remove no more than 1cm (½in).

When to cut a baby's hair

Baby hair is very fine and soon starts to look a little 'raggy'. If the ends are trimmed every 6–8 weeks it will keep the hair looking tidy. There's no right or wrong time for a baby to have a first hair cut, but hair should be trimmed before it gets near the eyes.

CHOOSING A HAIRBRUSH

A well-made brush should last for many years. All brushes should have even tufts or rows of bristles to allow loose, shed hairs to collect in the grooves without interfering with the action of the brush.

There are many types of hairbrush available, and they fall into two main categories – those for everyday brushing and those for styling.

A natural bristle is recommended for general use because it has a more gentle action and redistributes the natural hair oils evenly.

For styling – usually done using a hair dryer – brushes tend to be made of nylon. It is best to choose a brush with rounded nylon ball tips that are moulded as part of the bristle and not just attached to the top, because they easily break off. Using a brush that is missing the nylon ball tips can scratch the scalp or damage the hair.

Thick coarse hair can benefit from using a paddle brush which can create a smooth look and style. If you have wavy hair look for a round vented brush. To avoid frizziness, curly hair should be 'brushed' with a wide-tooth comb, while a vented brush with natural bristles is ideal for thin, fine hair. Long hair should be detangled with a wide-tooth comb first, before being styled.

To clean your brush use a comb to remove built up hair. Soak the brush in hot water and a few drops of shampoo. Rinse and dry thoroughly.

Brushing your hair

Always start brushing in sections from the ends of the hair working up to the roots. Hold the mesh of hair just above the section being brushed. This reduces tension on the hair strands and will prevent breakage.

100 strokes a night?
Women used to brush their hair 100 times each night to remove dirt and disperse natural oils. This is no longer necessary, but it can still be beneficial: use a natural bristle brush and brush deeply from the scalp.

Body hair

As mammals, all human beings have body hair. The amount varies with genetic background and age – whether it is too much or too little is a matter of personal perception and social norms.

The amount of body hair in some areas is a major source of concern for many people, who can spend significant amounts of time and money trying to remove it.

REMOVING UNWANTED HAIR

The most common methods of hair removal fall into two categories:

- **Epilation** This means that the hair is removed below the surface of the skin, and refers to the complete removal of the hair from the follicle. This can be done by plucking, waxing or sugaring.
- **Depilation** This is removal at skin level, either by chemically damaging the hairs so that they break off, or by shaving.

Epilation

Waxing, sugaring and plucking are painful but successful ways of removing hair. The effect is temporary (usually no more than six weeks, and often considerably less) since new hair cells continue to be produced by the follicle. Repeated removal of hairs can cause disruption of the anatomy of the hair growing area and lead to the formation of ingrowing hairs and inflammation of the follicles (folliculitis). These conditions are difficult to treat.

Plucking is viable for small areas, but it is too painful and time-consuming for larger areas. Plucking is ideal for any stray hairs, but avoid over-plucking eyebrows, as the hairs may not grow back.

Wax can be applied hot or cold, and is a home or salon treatment. It involves the application of wax to areas of unwanted hair. After the wax hardens it is pulled off the skin along with the embedded hairs. Generally, waxing done by someone else is more successsful than self-administered – partly due to training, but also because people find it hard to inflict discomfort on themselves. Sugaring uses the same technique, but uses a sugar solution to adhere to the hairs instead of wax.

Depilation

If epilation seems too uncomfortable, depilatory cream may be the answer. Again this is a temporary solution, since the hair follicle is not being damaged and hair will regrow. Depilation creams are easy to apply and work by removing hair just below the surface of the skin. They contain sodium thioglycolate and calcium thioglycolate, which dissolve the keratin chemically. The mixture of chemicals produces an unpleasant odour, but this goes after rinsing. The disadvantages are that the effect is shortlived, often less than a week, and the chemicals can irritate the skin. They should not be used on sensitive areas such as the face, and if a cream is being used for the first time it should be patch tested first to avoid an adverse reaction.

Before applying the cream wash the area with a warm face flannel to soften the hairs and open the follicles

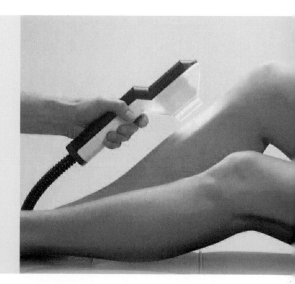

LASER HAIR REMOVAL

Laser hair removal works by pulsing a laser for a millisecond, emitting a beam of light onto the skin. The light energy passes harmlessly through the skin, but is absorbed by the pigment in the hair follicle and hair shaft. By absorbing this laser energy, the hair follicles are disabled, impairing their ability to grow.

Treatment is described as being a little uncomfortable – a tingling, stinging sensation. As some areas of the body are more sensitive than others, topical anaesthetic may be applied before treatment to lessen discomfort. The treatment time depends on the area: the upper lip takes only a few minutes while the back or legs can take up to an hour.

Laser hair removal works best on people with fair skin and dark hair: blonde, grey and white hairs do not respond well, although a lot depends on the skill of the practitioner you choose. Treatments are scheduled to coincide with hair follicles being in an active growth phase – which is every 4 to 8 weeks. Laser hair removal is often termed 'permanent'; most people lose up to 70 per cent of hair after three to five treatments.

so the cream will penetrate better. An effective chemical depilatory will damage the skin as well as the hair, but in normal healthy skin this does not usually cause a problem. Do not leave the cream on longer than recommended.

Shaving

Shaving is even faster than using a depilatory cream. Women have the same choices as men in terms of wet or dry shaving; both are equally fast and efficient.

• **Wet shaving** Although more time-consuming, this causes fewer problems of dry skin and chafing than dry shaving. Modern shaving creams contain moisturisers and the action of rubbing in cream tones the skin. In ancient times oil was used to soften the beard prior to shaving, and recently this method has been reintroduced. Wet shaving provides the closest shave.

• **Dry shaving** The obvious advantage of the dry shave is that it dispenses with the need for hot water and shaving cream, allowing shaving to be cleaner, safer and more mobile. Electric shavers make it virtually impossible to cut yourself. Dry shaving typically does not produce as close a shave as wet shaving. Different areas of the body should be shaved in different directions:

• The face should be shaved first in the direction of hair growth and then against.

• Legs should be shaved in an upward direction, against the direction of hair growth.

• Underarm hair grows in different directions, so this area should be shaved down, up and then across for the closest shave.

• Bikini area skin is very delicate, so hair should be shaved in the same direction as hair growth to prevent irritation.

FEMALE FACIAL HAIR

For many women, excessive or over-dark facial hair is a particular cause of embarrassment and concern. A number of treatments are available, both temporary and permanent.

Bleaching the hair with dilute hydrogen peroxide and ammonia solution is a safe and simple way of disguising hair growth. If using a product for the first time, always patch test your skin beforehand. Shaving should be avoided in this area as it can leave unsightly stubble. However, waxing is effective, leaving the skin clean and smooth. It is best to visit a beauty therapist for this.

In skilled hands, electrolysis and short-wave diathermy can successfully destroy individual hairs. Electrolysis is a long process and can cause local pain. Unwanted effects may be pitted scars and post-inflammatory hyperpigmentation (PIHP). Re-growth occurs but gradually the hairs become thinner and paler. It is vital to find a reputable practitioner, as poorly done electrolysis can cause scarring.

UNWANTED MALE NOSE AND EAR HAIR

It is thought that the male hormone reponsible for baldness may also be linked to nasal and ear hair growth – as men get older this hair becomes longer and coarser. Ear and nose hair can be easily trimmed, but it should never be plucked, as this could tear the delicate skin and cause an infection. The safest method is to use a specially designed electric trimmer.

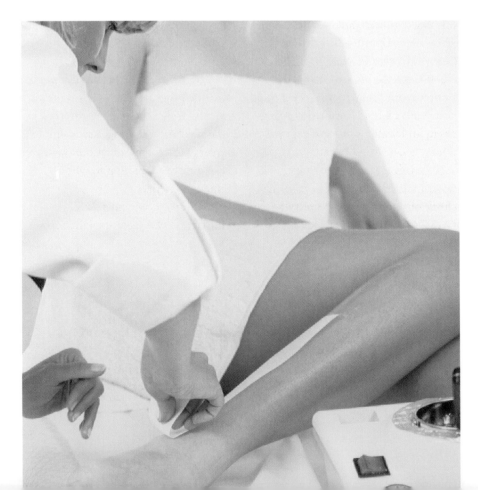

Smooth operator
To avoid prolonging the localised pain of waxing, strips should be pulled upwards quickly, in a single motion.

Healthy and good-looking nails

Many of us do not give our nails a lot of thought. However, since they protect our fingers and toes and enhance our touch and fine motor skills, their health is extremely important.

NORMAL NAIL GROWTH

Fingernails grow at a rate of about 0.1mm a day and are replaced approximately every 4–6 months. Toenails grow more slowly and can take up to twice as long to replace themselves. How quickly and how well they grow depends on several factors: age, hormones, time of year (they grow faster in the summer), infections, nutrition and trauma.

Each nail rises up from a nail root made up of the normal layers of cells in the skin. The outer layer forms the cuticle and the nail itself rests on what is called the nail bed. The nail bed supports the nail as it grows outward from the nail matrix. It normally reaches the end of the nail bed and extends beyond it: when it does so, this portion is termed the free edge.

WHY NAILS BREAK

Nails can break, tear or split for many different reasons. The most common reason is having the nails submerged in water and detergents too much. It is important to protect the nails from excessive moisture as this can cause splitting and peeling. The easy answer to this is to wear household gloves while doing chores, especially washing up and gardening. Try to avoid nail damage – don't use your nails as tools for prising things open, and watch out for closing doors: it pays to take care.

If, however, you know that this is not a major factor in your case then check out your diet and lifestyle (see page 72). You might be lacking in nutrients that will not only benefit your nails but will also do wonders for your skin and hair.

HOW TO CUT NAILS

The best time for cutting your nails is after a bath when your nails are softer and so easier to cut. This is particularly the case with toenails.

Helping hands
It is important to protect the skin on the hands as it has extensive contact with cleaning agents and environmental hazards.

A proper nail clipper will take most of the effort out of cutting and is more controllable than scissors.

Take care not to cut your nails too short as this can expose extremely sensitive skin, normally protected by the nail. After cutting, use a simple emery file to even them out, always filing in one direction for the smoothest effect.

Similarly, don't cut toenails too short. Cut them straight across to prevent ingrown toenails. Smooth them off so that they do not scratch your skin or get caught – or make holes – in your socks or tights.

If you find bending over a problem, either due to a sore hip or pregnancy, there are long-handled toenail clippers on the market, which will make the job much easier.

Do nail strengtheners work?

Nail strengtheners do make nails harder, but there are a couple of things to bear in mind. They seem to work best when you use them for relatively short periods of time. Experts recommend you do not use them for any longer than 6–8 weeks at a time. Continuous use will over harden your nails, making them brittle, so that you have turned one nail problem into another.

When choosing a nail strengthener be sure to get a product that does not contain formaldehyde; this toxic substance was once widely used, but has now been superceded by safer ingredients. Take extra care during pregnancy: if you have any doubts over a product's safety, don't use it.

ASK THE EXPERT

GIVE YOURSELF A MANICURE
You will need:
- *a bowl of warm water*
- *nail clippers*
- *emery board*
- *cuticle pusher (wooden or plastic, or use a cottonbud)*
- *scrub cream*
- *hand cream*

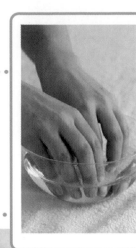

Wash your hands and clean out any dirt under your fingernails, then soak your nails in warm water for about 5 minutes; this will soften both the nails and cuticles.

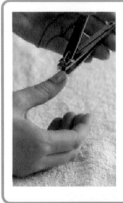

Clip your nails to the desired length and shape, finishing by filing them to smooth the edge. Take care to file in one direction only to 'seal' the edge instead of roughing it up.

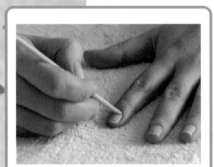

Gently push back the cuticle. Do not damage the cuticles as they protect the nail bed from trauma and bacteria. Only cut a piece of cuticle away if it is in danger of tearing.

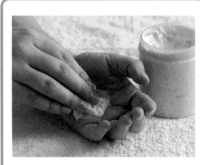

Take a generous amount of scrub cream (a facial one is fine) and massage this into your hands for a few minutes: this will remove any dead skin cells. Rinse well to leave rosy, smooth skin.

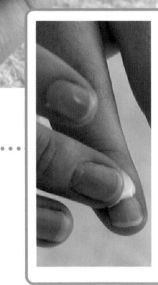

Thoroughly dry your hands then apply hand cream, making sure you don't forget to massage it into the cuticles to keep them supple and to prevent them from cracking.

Cutting babies' nails

It can be daunting cutting an infant's nails. As a baby's nails are so soft, however, initially you may find that they flake away all by themselves and you don't need to cut them. A lot of parents nibble off tiny nails to prevent having to take clippers or scissors to them. Once this becomes too difficult, do what you would do yourself. Wait until after a bath and use small nail clippers to cut away any nails that are too long and may be causing self-inflicted scratches. Try to prevent cutting away too much, as this will only cause discomfort to the baby, especially if the nail should become infected. Trimming little and often is the best option.

NAIL CONDITION

Nails in a poor condition can be a result of dietary deficiencies (see page 72). A crash diet or a strict vegan lifestyle can also affect nail health. Contrary to popular belief, white spots on the nails have nothing to do with calcium deficiency; they are simply little air pockets under the surface, usually caused by minor traumas to the nail.

Vertical ridges on nails are a normal sign of ageing which start to occur in middle age. They can't be prevented, but they can be smoothed out by buffing. Horizontal ridges, also known as 'Beau's lines', are caused by an interruption in the growth of the nail due to recent illness, severe stress, or injury to the nail – these ridges grow out in time.

FOOD AND DRINK FOR SKIN, HAIR AND NAILS

So much of our appearance is determined by our internal health. For glowing skin, shiny hair and strong nails your diet needs to contain a range of essential nutrients, particularly those which contribute to the structure of collagen in the skin and keratin in the nails and hair.

 66 *For overall nail, skin and hair health, each meal should be nutritious and well-balanced. Here are some meal ideas to try.*

 68 *The skin directly reflects our health. These are the essential vitamins or minerals you need to keep dull and tired looking skin at bay.*

 71 *Shiny hair and strong nails depend on a good supply of iron, zinc and calcium: the best sources of these nutrients are described here.*

Eating plan for healthy skin, hair and nails

A diet consisting of fresh, unprocessed foods is vital for the health of your entire body, not just your skin. Try to include plenty of fresh fruit and vegetables and foods with high levels of essential fatty acids.

Breakfast

1 bowl of muesli with
semi-skimmed milk, topped with
a tablespoon of flaxseeds and
a handful of raspberries
1 cup of herbal tea
  OR
half a grapefruit
1 pot of low-fat yoghurt topped
with a tablespoon of flaxseeds
1 slice of toast with 1 tsp low-fat
spread and 1 tsp yeast extract
1 cup of herbal tea

Lunch

Grilled chicken breast served with
young leaf spinach salad with tofu
dressing, and ciabatta bread
Sliced mango
Glass of water or calcium-fortified
soya milk

OR

1 portion of smoked mackerel served
with a potato salad made using
low-fat yoghurt and Dijon mustard,
and a portion of cherry tomatoes
Orange and date salad
Glass of water or orange juice

Flaxseeds are a rich source of essential fatty acids including omega-3, 6 and 9.

Dinner

Pan-seared salmon fillet served with baked sweet potatoes and stir-fried courgettes and mixed peppers.
Mixed fruit salad topped with Greek-style yoghurt
1 cup of green tea
   OR
Grilled pork chop served with apple sauce, home-made gravy, blanched broccoli and carrots, and mashed potatoes
Baked apple with a handful of sultanas, served with home-made custard made using skimmed milk
1 cup of herbal tea

Snacks

A handful of pumpkin seeds
Raw vegetables with low-fat hummous
Unlimited fruit
Rye bread topped with low-fat cream cheese and sliced pineapple

Remember to drink plenty of water throughout the day to prevent dehydration.

How foods affect the skin

Just as foods can affect energy levels, they can also affect appearance. A balanced intake of nutrients will contribute to your health on the inside, and will be reflected on the outside in clear skin, strong nails and healthy hair.

NUTRIENTS FOR HEALTHY SKIN

The most important vitamins and minerals for the health of your skin are vitamin A, the B vitamins, vitamin C, vitamin E and zinc.

Vitamin A

Vitamin A helps to maintain the structural integrity of skin cells. A deficiency disturbs the delicate balance of the skin and results in the loss of cells that produce lubricants to keep the skin soft and supple. This in turn leads to infection, irritation and sloughing off of the surface of the skin.

Everyday foods contain two forms of vitamin A: retinol, which is derived from animal products, and carotenes (mostly beta-carotene), which can be found in fruit and vegetables. The best sources of retinol are liver, fish liver oils, kidneys, dairy foods and eggs. Beta-carotene is found mainly in carrots and dark green, yellow or orange vegetables. The darker the vegetable, the more beta-carotene it contains. The daily recommended amount (DRA) of vitamin A is 700µg for a man and 600µg for a woman. A glass of carrot juice or a 90g serving of spinach provides the daily amount; a serving of liver or liver pâté exceeds it at least four-fold.

B-group vitamins

Niacin is a B vitamin, and a deficiency has been linked to a disease called pellagra. Symptoms include dermatitis, where the skin becomes dark and scaly – especially when exposed to light – as well as diarrhoea and dementia. Although it is rare to develop a deficiency in the

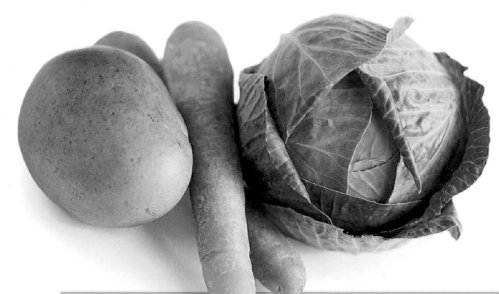

Skin-smart diet
The first step towards a better complexion is to ensure you are not missing vital nutrients in your diet. Fruit and vegetables are packed with skin-boosting vitamins and minerals.

VITAMIN A CONTENT OF SELECTED FOODS

	Portion size (g)	Vitamin A (µg)		Portion size (g)	Vitamin A (µg)
Liver, calf, fried	100	25200	Spinach, boiled	90	576
Liver, pig, stewed	100	22600	Curly kale	95	534
Liver, lamb, fried	100	19700	Mango	140	450
Liver, chicken, fried	100	10500	Carrots, young, boiled	60	443
Liver pâté	40	2960	Spring greens, boiled	95	359
Sweet potato, baked	130	1112	Butternut squash, baked	65	354
Carrots, old, boiled	60	756	Cantaloupe melon	100	322
Carrot juice	60	678	Paw paw	140	189
Swiss chard, boiled	50	655	Savoy cabbage, boiled	95	100

UK, it makes sense to ensure an adequate amount in the diet. The DRA of niacin is 17mg for a man and 13mg for a woman. Good sources include meat, potatoes, bread and fortified breakfast cereals.

Deficiency of B-group vitamins riboflavin (vitamin B_2) and pyridoxine (vitamin B_6) cause skin lesions or sores, especially at the corners of the mouth, eyelids and genital areas. Deficiency is rare unless the diet is short on milk, meat, fortified cereal products and eggs. The DRAs of riboflavin and pyridoxine are 1.3mg and 1.4mg respectively for a man and 1.1mg and 1.2mg for a woman.

The B-group vitamin biotin is needed in small amounts by the body to break down fat. Rich sources include offal and egg yolk, while smaller amounts are found in milk and dairy products, cereals, fish, yeast, fruit and vegetables. Biotin deficiency is rare. It can occur if excessive amounts of raw egg white are consumed. Raw egg white contains the compound avidin which attaches or binds itself to biotin making it unavailable to the body for absorption. In such cases, deficiency leads to a dry scaly dermatitis.

Vitamin C

Vitamin C is an important antioxidant helping to maintain healthy tissues and to fight wrinkles. It also plays an important role in the formation of collagen in the skin. A deficiency results in bleeding, especially from blood vessels underneath the surface of the skin and the gums. The best sources include citrus fruits, potatoes, peppers, cabbage and courgettes. The DRA is 40mg for all adults.

Vitamin E

Vitamin E is another important antioxidant for healthy skin. It helps to maintain the structural integrity of cell membranes. This vitamin occurs widely in foods and, because it is fat soluble, can be stored in the body, so deficiency is rare. The richest sources are vegetable oils, nuts and seeds, some cereal products and egg yolk. The DRA is 7mg per adult – cooking with 1 tablespoon of sunflower oil and eating a handful of hazelnuts provides the daily requirement.

Zinc

Zinc works with vitamin C to make healthy collagen – an essential component of connective tissues. The total amount of zinc in the adult body has been estimated to be around 1.4 to 2.3g, of which 20 per cent is in the skin. A deficiency can lead to weeping dermatitis around the body orifices and on the extremities such as hands and feet, eczema, poor wound healing and reduced immune system function. Zinc deficiency has also been shown to worsen pre-existing acne. Oysters, pumpkin seeds, pecan nuts, red meat, wholewheat and rye flour are all good sources. The DRA is 9.5mg for a man and 7.0mg for a woman.

Essential fatty acids (EFAs)

Some types of polyunsaturated fat are termed essential because they must be derived from the diet – the body cannot make them from other polyunsaturated fats. These EFAs are called omega-3 and omega-6 fats, and they help to hydrate the skin and increase its moisture content. A deficiency of EFAs can result in a scaly rash because water loss from the skin increases. Topical

Do EFAs offer relief from eczema and psoriasis?

The incidence of atopic eczema has been rising over the past decade. Many hypotheses have been suggested, including a decline in breastfeeding and a deficiency of essential fatty acids (EFAs). Studies have shown conflicting results; some have concluded that breastfeeding prevents atopic eczema, whilst others have found no evidence. Similarly with EFAs, trials using fish oil as a dietary supplement for atopic eczema have shown conflicting results, although the EFA linoleic acid (found in evening primrose oil and starfruit oil) has been shown to be beneficial for eczema.

The effect of EFAs on psoriasis appears to be more positive. A number of trials using fish oil supplements to treat psoriasis showed positive results, but again these are inconclusive.

ASK THE EXPERT

applications on the skin have been shown to reverse these symptoms.

Good sources of EFAs include oily fish, vegetables and red meat. A healthy eating recommendation is a daily intake of omega-3 fats of 0.2g a day. This can be achieved by eating one to two servings of oily fish a week. Other sources include flaxseeds and flaxseed oils. Flaxseeds are available from health food shops and can be sprinkled on salads and cooked vegetables, or combined with flour to make breads and pancakes. Flaxseed oil comes in an edible form and, like olive and rapeseed oils, is high in unsaturated fats which is heart healthy. It also contains lignans which have anti-cancer properties.

FOOD ALLERGIES

The immune system protects the body from harmful foreign proteins called antigens by generating a response to get rid of them. Antibodies are produced, which specifically bind with the antigen to deactivate and eliminate it. In food allergies an individual's immune system reacts in this way to a food which has no harmful effect in the majority of people.

Signs and symptoms of food allergy vary from person to person. There are different types of reaction and one of the most common kinds involves the production of histamine, which can cause a number of symptoms including urticaria or skin rash. Such allergies have been linked to the consumption of milk, egg, fish, shellfish, nuts and strawberries in certain individuals, and if any one of these is implicated exclusion of that food is advised. This type of allergy arises in early childhood and appears trigger abnormal inflammatory processes in the skin which are chronic and recurrent.

DIGESTION AND THE SKIN

An important aspect of skin health is a healthy colon and digestive process. If the colon is not moving food efficiently, or the liver or kidneys are struggling to process waste, this can lead to a build-up of toxins in the bloodstream. This may have an impact on the appearance of the skin.

To aid the proper functioning of the digestive system it is important to get plenty of fibre in the diet. You should also limit the amount of processed foods and sugars in the diet and limit alcohol intake. A well-balanced diet goes a long way to maintaining skin health. Many people find that drinking a cup of warm water with a squeeze of fresh lemon juice first thing in the morning helps to flush out toxins, while herbalists recommend milk thistle supplements to help cleanse the liver and improve skin health.

Drink your way to skin health
Drinking more water could be the simple tonic your skin needs. Water acts as an internal moisturiser, promoting clearer skin and a glowing complexion.

IT'S NOT TRUE!

'Fatty foods cause acne'

Scientific studies have not found a connection between diet and acne. However, because acne is caused by an increase in the production of sebum – a natural oil – it is often thought that fatty foods are responsible. This is not true – chocolates, crisps and other fatty foods do not cause acne. Some people also believe that acne is due to poor hygiene. Again, this is untrue and vigorous washing and scrubbing can make acne worse. Another myth states that acne must be left to run its course. The truth is, acne can be cleared up. If acne products haven't worked, consider seeing a dermatologist: sufferers don't have to endure acne or develop scars from it.

WATER – VITAL FOR SKIN HEALTH

Water is essential for life; it makes up around two-thirds of body weight and is vital for regulating body fluids. The average adult should consume 2.5 litres of water a day. This will ensure that you avoid dehydration, which can lead to dull, lifeless and dry skin.

MALNUTRITION

Although rarely seen in Westernised countries, malnutrition can lead to a skin condition in which a sequence of changes similar to sunburn occur. The skin becomes darker, with the outer skin becoming dry and thin, and easily split and ulcerated.

Foods for healthy hair and nails

Eat a well-balanced diet for the general good health of your hair and nails, with particular emphasis on keeping iron, calcium and zinc levels up. Dietary deficiency is one among several different causes of hair loss and problem nails.

IRON

Better known for keeping blood in good health, iron also has an effect on the condition of your hair. General hair loss has been linked to low iron stores, which means that women who have heavy periods, or who eat little or no red meat, have an increased risk of hair loss.

To maximise iron absorption, various dietary factors should be considered when preparing meals.

- Consuming vitamin C-rich foods such as fruits, vegetables and juice with a meal will double or treble the amount of iron absorbed from non-meat or fish sources.
- Protein-rich foods such as meat, fish and seafood promote the absorption of iron.

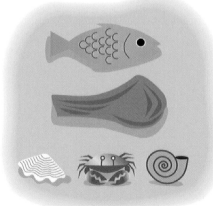

- Phytate and fibre-rich foods such as cereals, bran, seeds and nuts inhibit the absorption of iron.
- Tea, coffee, cocoa, spinach and spices contain compounds called phenols which will inhibit iron absorption from pulses, legumes, cereals and vegetables.

- Calcium-rich foods such as milk and cheese interfere with the absorption of iron in a meal.
- Fermented products such as soy sauce, enhance the absorption of iron from non-meat or fish sources.

To optimise iron levels or to replenish your body's stores, include iron-rich foods in your diet. The best sources are red meat – especially liver – egg yolks, dried fruit, fortified breakfast cereals and green leafy vegetables. Then, to maximise iron absorption, eat these foods together with those that are high in vitamins. For example, have a glass of orange juice with your meal. Try not to drink tea or coffee for at least half an hour after a meal to minimise the adverse effect of tea, coffee and milk on iron absorption.

Our requirements for iron vary throughout our lives: adolescent girls and adult women need 14.8mg per day, whilst adolescent boys need 11.3mg per day and adult men require 8.7mg per day. Female requirements are higher because of menstrual losses.

THE NEED FOR ZINC

Zinc is an essential component of hair – scalp hair in children has been estimated to contain 125–225µg zinc per gram of hair. In some studies zinc deficiency has been shown to lead to hair loss, excessive fragility of hair, sparse scalp hair and absent pubic hair. Zinc deficiency has been shown to be the cause of hair loss in the disease acrodermatitis enteropathica, which is characterised by alopecia as well as diarrhoea and dermatitis. Hair is lost diffusely and extensively and existing hair lacks pigment, making it fragile and prone to excessive breakage.

Although zinc can be found in a wide variety of foods, its absorption by the body depends on the composition of the diet. The risk of zinc deficiency is highest when the diet contains large quantities of unrefined cereals and little animal protein.

- **Phytates** in wholegrain cereals, legumes and other vegetables, bind to zinc, making it unavailable for absorption by the body.
- **Animal protein** improves the absorption of zinc from foods.
- **Essential fatty acid (EFA)** deficiency has been shown to cause hair loss. EFAs form two groups – omega-3 and omega-6 fats – and can be found in oily fish, as well as in vegetables and red meat.

MALNUTRITION

Malnutrition can have a very serious effect on hair, weakening its attachment to the skin so that it plucks out easily and painlessly. Remaining hair becomes thin and straight and may turn grey. Patients can go completely bald, although this is usually reversible.

FOODS FOR HEALTHY NAILS

Nails are a type of skin, made up mainly of the protein keratin. They grow at the rate of around 0.05 to 1.2mm a week. Our nails reveal a great deal about the state of our health. There are numerous vitamins and minerals that are specifically needed by the body to make healthy and strong nails, so deficiencies over a period of time will have a detrimental effect.

Iron is essential for the maintenance of healthy cells, and a long-term deficiency can cause nails to become spoon shaped, brittle and thin. Two sources of iron – haem and non-haem – can be found in our foods, and there are various ways of making sure iron is absorbed when we eat (see page 71).

Very small amounts of the B-group vitamin biotin are needed for the formation of strong nails. This can be produced by the bacteria which live in our large intestine. Rich sources include egg yolk, milk and dairy products, liver and other organ meats, soy products and yeast.

Calcium is the most abundant mineral in the body, with about 99 per cent of it occuring in the bones, teeth and nails. When bound together with phosphorous, calcium strengthens the skeleton. Few foods contain significant amounts of calcium besides milk, yoghurt, cheese, most breads, calcium-fortified soya milk, tofu, green leafy vegetables and hard water.

The DRA for calcium for an adult is 700mg a day, which is achieved, for example, by eating a pot of yoghurt, a small chunk of cheese and a portion of young leaf spinach. Breastfeeding mothers require an additional 550mg a day: to meet this add a portion of tofu and a slice of white bread, for example, or a portion of canned sardines with bones and a handful of sultanas.

CALCIUM CONTENT OF SELECTED FOODS

	Portion	Calcium (mg)
Sardines with bones, canned in brine	140g	540
Whole-milk yoghurt	150g	300
Cheddar	40g	288
Low-fat yoghurt	150g	285
Cheddar, vegetarian	40g	276
Semi skimmed/ or skimmed milk	150ml	175
Whole milk	150ml	168
Brie cheese	50g	92
Ice cream, dairy	125g	90
Fromage frais	100g	89
Baked beans, canned in tomato sauce	135g	65
White bread	36g	40
Watercress	20g	34
White rice, boiled	180g	32
Boiled egg	50g	29
Cabbage, white, boiled	95g	25
Peanuts, dry roasted	40g	21
Courgettes, boiled	100g	19
Wholemeal bread	36g	19
Sultanas	18g	12
Braising steak, stewed	140g	11
Potatoes, boiled	175g	9
Apples	100g	4
Cod, baked	120g	3

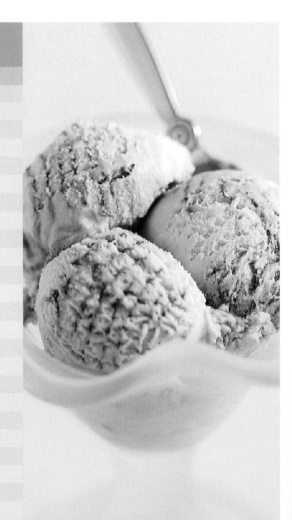

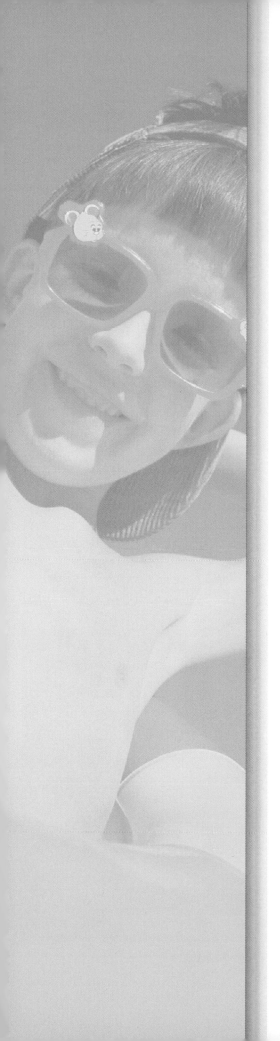

THE WEATHER AND YOUR SKIN

Most people are now aware that despite the good things the sun can do for skin and general health, it can also cause damage if we do not take precautions. Other weather factors such as wind rain and snow may also have an impact on our skin, hair and nails.

 74   *Safety in the sun is of paramount importance for everyone, especially for children, to keep skin young-looking and free from disease.*

 81   *In some circumstances winter can pose as many risks to skin health as summer does: find out how to minimise their impact.*

How the sun affects your skin

In the UK about 34,000 people are diagnosed with skin cancer every year. Incidence has risen rapidly over the past 50 years and it is now the second most common cancer. Increased exposure to sun is a major cause of this rise.

ALL ABOUT SUN

Sunlight is essential for human well-being. Not only does it make us feel good, it also produces heat and illumination, and through plant photosynthesis, the food necessary for our survival. The sun is also our primary source of vitamin D, essential for bone health.

Sunlight contains radiation of many different wavelengths, from invisible low-frequency infra-red heat radiation, through the visible light spectrum, to invisible ultra-violet rays. Shorter wavelength X-rays also form part of sunlight.

What is UVR?

The light rays of ultra-violet radiation (UVR) are categorised into three different wavebands, called A, B and C.

The sun is our principal source of UVR, although artificial sources can be significant for people such as welders and some hospital workers. Outdoor workers have up to four times the total UVR exposure of indoor workers. Although low-intensity fluorescent lights may be a source of UVR for indoor workers, this has not yet been proved.

Outdoor activities such as sport and gardening also increase the level of daily UVR exposure.

What increases the amount of radiation?

UV radiation is reflected and altered by different surfaces, and damage can be greater under certain circumstances. Exposure is increased at high altitude, at low latitude and nearer the equator. UV rays are strongest during the summer. Reflection of UVR is increased 25 per cent by sand, and 5 per cent by water. Reflection is lessened by cloud cover (20–90 per cent) and the passage of light through water. It is unaffected by heat, cold, wind and visible light.

For the last few decades, scientists have been monitoring changes in the ozone layer – the protective layer of the stratosphere. Due to damage caused by human activities, ozone levels have been reduced. This has lead to an increase in the levels of UVB rays reaching the earth.

UVR AND THE SKIN

Two types of UV effect are felt by the skin: acute effects, which appear within a few hours – such as vitamin D production, tanning or sunburn – or chronic effects which are cumulative and may not appear for years – such as photoageing or skin cancer. The only non-damaging effect of UVR on the skin is the production of vitamin D.

SKIN TYPES

Knowing your skin type is a useful way to predict how your skin will react to the sun. The types below are used by dermatologists to treat skin diseases such as psoriasis with UV light. People with types I to II need extra care when deciding how much exposure they can tolerate and how quickly they will respond to treatment.

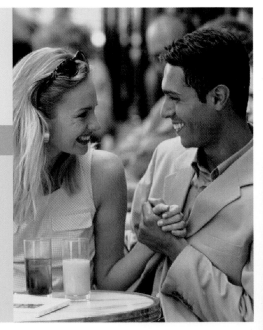

SKIN TYPE	SUN REACTION	TANNING	TYPICAL COMPLEXION
I	always burns	never	very fair
II	often burns	tans lightly	fair
III	sometimes burns	tans progressively	fair/medium
IV	rarely burns	tans easily	olive
V	rarely burns	tans deeply	Asian
VI	never burns	tans deeply	Afro-Caribbean

UVA rays pass effortlessly through the ozone layer and they make up the majority of our sun exposure.

Most UVB rays are absorbed by the ozone layer, but enough pass through to cause damage.

UVC rays are the most dangerous but fortunately are blocked by the ozone layer and don't reach the earth.

VITAMIN D

Vitamin D is formed when UV light converts 7-dehydrocholesterol in the skin into vitamin D_3. A protein in the skin then transports it to the blood and the liver for use.

TANNING

The skin has various mechanisms to protect itself against the harmful effects of the sun.

When the skin is exposed to sunlight, melanin in the epidermis is redistributed towards the surface to absorb the UVA rays. A slight darkening of the skin, called immediate pigment tanning, is seen. However, this is only temporary and fades 3–36 hours after exposure.

A second process called delayed tanning occurs when the skin is exposed to UVB rays. More melanocytes are produced and melanin production is increased, causing the skin to appear darker. The tough outer layer of the skin also thickens to absorb more of the UVB radiation. This two-part process takes one or more days and produces a noticeable tan that can last for weeks or even months.

This thickening and tanning provides some protection against further UV damage, but can make the skin more vulnerable to cancer.

WHAT IS SUNBURN?

Sunburn is an inflammatory redness of the skin, caused by overexposure to UV radiation, particularly UVB. It is a sign of severe cellular damage. The small blood vessels in the skin dilate and increase the blood flow to the skin's surface making it red and painful. UVB damage to the DNA of skin cells triggers several inflammatory pathways, causing a swelling of the skin.

A sunburn appears two hours after exposure, and develops over the next 24 hours. The skin turns red and blisters, several days later the dead skin cells peel off. In severe cases, the burn may occur with sunstroke.

IMMUNOSUPPRESSION

UVR damage to DNA triggers the release of suppressor T-lymphocytes in the skin. These reduce immune response, and subsequently increase the risk of infection or skin cancer.

PHOTOAGEING

The damaging effects of UVA can be seen in the premature ageing and wrinkling of chronically sun-exposed skin. Collagen and elastin fibres lose

UVR intensity
Levels of UVR vary depending on the time of day, time of year, altitude and distance from the equator. UV rays are most intense during midday hours in the summer, although they are always present, even in winter.

their elasticity and appear thickened and clumped. This accounts for the leathery appearance of exposed skin. Photoaged skin also shows epidermal thinning and irregular pigmentation.

SKIN CANCER

UV damages the genes which can lead to cells losing their normal growth control system. The immune system then fails to identify the abnormal cells, and cancer develops. There are three forms of skin cancer related to sun exposure. Malignant melanoma is linked to sporadic but intense sun exposure, particularly sunburn in childhood. Squamous cell carcinoma and basal cell carcinoma are more treatable, and are thought to be linked to more life-long low-grade exposure to UVR.

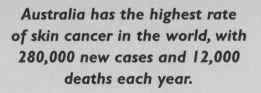

Australia has the highest rate of skin cancer in the world, with 280,000 new cases and 12,000 deaths each year.

WHY DO WE WANT A TAN?

A hundred years ago the idea that a tan could be desirable would have seemed absurd. In countries where most people were fair-skinned, tans were associated with people who worked outdoors and were a badge of low social status.

Attitudes started to change in the 1920s when Coco Chanel introduced the tan as a fashion accessory. At the same time artificial sun rays began to be used to treat some skin diseases. So being brown came to mean being healthy. After the Second World War foreign travel became more desirable and affordable, and a tan was seen as a sign of affluence.

However, even the lightest tan is a sign of skin damage. The rate at which people burn in the sun varies and this determines skin type. Skin types I and II have fewer melanocytes and tend to burn easily.

Attitudes are now changing as evidence mounts of the damage the sun can do, but many people still seek a 'perfect tan'. The safest tan is a fake one. There is a wide range of products available to produce a fake tan in a few hours.

SUN PROTECTION

Protection from the sun is extremely important, particularly for children. Since the 1980s Australians have grown up with a public health programme – known as 'Slip, slop, slap' – which advocates:

- **Slipping** on a (long-sleeved close-weave) shirt.
- **Slopping** on the sunscreen regularly, especially after swimming.
- **Slapping** on a hat that will shade the neck.

This is sensible advice for everyone.

How sunscreens work

Sunscreens contain organic chemical compounds that absorb UV radiation and sunblocks contain finely ground particles that reflect UVR away from the skin. They are available in many forms, including ointments, creams, gels, lotions, sprays and wax sticks.

All sunscreens are labelled with a sun protection factor (SPF) number which tells you how long you can stay in the sun before you burn. If you would normally burn in 30 minutes, a factor 20 SPF sunscreen will enable you to prolong that to 20 x 30 minutes. Most recommendations nowadays are that it is not worth using a sunscreen with an SPF of less than 15, or you will be applying suncream all day.

The factor only applies to UVB radiation, although some manufacturers also attempt to quantify UVA protection. It is also not a good idea to assume that you are safe for hours, simply because you are wearing a sunscreen: damage is cumulative, and it is never a good idea to be on a beach during the peak sun hours of around noon to 3pm. The American Academy of Dermatology recommends never deliberately sunbathing.

If you are going into the sun for more than 20 minutes you should use a sunscreen. Most people will

EXTRA SUN PRECAUTIONS FOR CHILDREN

Children need special protection from the sun. Even though skin cancer develops mainly in later life, it is our sun exposure as children that is probably most important in whether we develop it or not.

Severe sunburn before the age of 18 is a risk factor for malignant melanoma: one or more severe, blistering episodes of sunburn in childhood doubles the risk of skin cancer.

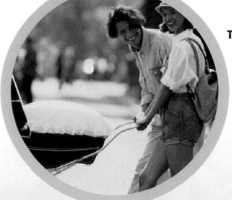

Total sun protection
Keep babies out of the sun completely, use high factor sunscreens, and cover them up.

Be clothing conscious
Make toddlers and older children wear a hat in the sun, and clothing that covers vulnerable skin, and limit the time they are out, especially during the hours of peak sun. Some fabrics are UV resistant and clothes made from these are a good choice.

Cool — and safe
Make children wear sunglasses with a UV filter to prevent cataract risk. Some 'fashion' sunglasses protect from UV, and some don't, so always check before buying.

Monitor SPF levels
Carry a credit-card sized SPF monitor with a photosensitive strip to tell you how strong the sun is.

77

HOLIDAYS AND SKIN PROBLEMS

Preventing skin problems on holiday is relatively easy as long as you are prepared. Before you go away check with your pharmacist whether any drugs you are taking might cause a phototoxic reaction in the sun. If they can, cover up and use high factor sunscreen. Most problems can be treated using the contents of a first-aid kit. Rarely, however, they may be more serious, so it is important to watch out for any serious reactions like spasms, shock or breathing difficulties. If these are present seek emergency medical help immediately.

USEFUL FIRST-AID ITEMS

Vinegar to pour on tentacles to prevent further release of toxins.
Baking soda a baking soda paste can help neutralise sting venom.
Antihistamines to ease the itch from bites, stings or prickly heat.
Paracetamol for fever or pain.
Witch hazel/aloe vera for burns, bites and general skin irritations.

Sunburn

Make sure that sun creams are applied for complete cover. If you miss parts of your body, oddly shaped areas of sunburn can appear, on your back or behind your ears, for example. Reapply sun cream after swimming.

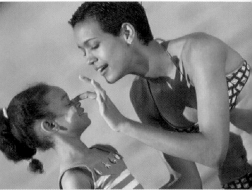

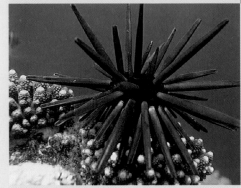

Bites and burrows

Larva nigrans The larvae from dog hookworm are excreted on the sand and can burrow into the skin, leaving a winding track on your leg or buttock. They move a few millimetres a day. The problem usually resolves spontaneously but drugs are available to cure the problem.

Sea urchin spines

If you develop painful lumps on the feet after a holiday abroad you may have unwittingly stepped on a sea urchin spine. These need to be removed by a minor operation before the lesions will settle down. It is good advice, therefore, to wear sandals while swimming.

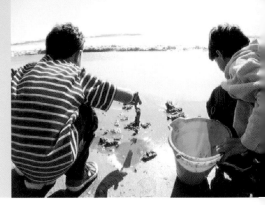

receive this amount of sun exposure daily, so it is good for your skin to use cosmetics that have daily use sunscreen in them. Even on a cloudy day there will be reflected UV light, so use it then as well.

- Sunscreen should be applied to dry skin at least 30 minutes before going outside, use liberal amounts so that it will penetrate the skin and not rub off immediately.
- A high factor sunscreen is no use if it washes off through swimming or sweating. 'Water-resistant'

sunscreen is less effective after 40 minutes in the water, and 'waterproof' after 80 minutes, so reapply regularly. If you have towelled dry, reapply sooner.

- Lips need cover, so use a sun-protective lip balm with SPF 15 or higher, or a sunblock.

Sunscreens are only effective for about two years after manufacture, after which they should be thrown away. The chemicals separate from the solution, so if your sunscreen feels gritty throw it out.

If you can't remember exactly when the sunscreen was bought, it would be safer to buy a new bottle than to risk inadequate sun protection. In some countries (though not the EU as yet) manufacturers are required to put production and use by dates on sunscreens, as for food products.

EMERGENCY TREATMENT FOR SUNBURN

The main symptoms of sunburn are pain and a sensation of heat in the affected skin, which can feel itchy

Insect bites

The severity of the reaction to insect bites varies from individual to individual. Most people get bitten but not all react. In malarial regions always be sure to take tablets to prevent malaria, and sleep under a mosquito net.

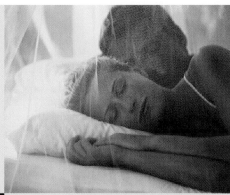

Sea bather's eruption

This is an itchy rash that comes up in the area covered by the swimsuit, and is caused by jellyfish and sea anemone larvae. It can be prevented by showering in fresh water after coming out of the sea.

Stings

Jellyfish stings produce itchy raised red bumps where tentacles touch the skin. If a tentacle is attached to the skin, use tweezers to remove it. *Weaver fish spines* protruding from the sand cause pain and redness when trodden on. Treat by putting the foot in warm water.

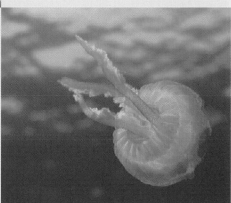

and tight. The skin may also be red, blistered or swollen. Some people develop shivering and a raised body temperature; they may also feel very weak. Peeling typically occurs about a week after the episode of burning.

Immediate treatment should include a spell in a cool bath, for at least 20 minutes, to try to remove some of the excess heat.

Avoiding dehydration is important. If you have been sweating a lot you may have lost a fair amount of body fluid, which must be replaced.

Aftersun creams or 1 per cent menthol-in-aqueous cream are soothing for mild sunburn. Paracetamol can reduce pain and fever, and topical steroids help to soothe inflamed skin.

SUNBEDS

Research suggests that as many as a fifth of British adults have used sunbeds at some time in their lives. The placing of these facilities in health clubs and gyms implies that this is a healthy thing to do, but this

> **We get about 80 per cent of our lifetime sun exposure before the age of 20.**

is far from the truth. Many people use them before a holiday, or have regular 'top ups' to maintain a tan after a holiday. Yet sunbeds can damage your skin for life.

They are designed to produce a tan by emitting UVA (some have a little UVB). UVA can cause premature ageing and also contribute to skin cancer. Sunbeds do not produce the thickening in skin that gradual natural exposure does, so using them before a holiday is not necessarily a protection against burning on holiday. The most important part of the body to protect is the eyes, so always use the mask provided. As little as 30 minutes a week over a period of years may cause increased fragility of the skin.

Sunbeds should not be used by the under 16s, by people with skin types I and II (see page 74), by anyone using photosensitive drugs (check the manufacturer's leaflet in the pack) or wearing cosmetics (wash before a session), or by anyone who has had skin cancer.

HOW SUN DAMAGES HAIR

Your hair may feel fried after a day at the beach, but hair can't get sunburnt because it is not living. Sun exposure damages the hair's natural protective film, as the scale-like cells that cover each individual hair begin to pull off. This will make hair feel fragile, dry, dull and brittle. Hair

Why is rainwater supposed to be good for washing?

When hard water dries on the skin it feels tight and dry, and this is compounded by the use of detergent-like soaps, bubble baths and shower gels. Rainwater is far softer than tap water in many parts of the UK, so the deposit left on the skin is reduced, as is the amount of soap necessary to produce lather.

Collecting rainwater for bathing is not really practical, so the best compromise is to avoid soap, using soap substitutes for washing, and moisturise regularly. If you have eczema it might be a good idea to have a water softening unit fitted to the washing machine, since the cotton and natural fibre clothing that help with eczema will respond better to washing in softened water, and also reduce the amount of washing powder and fabric softener needed.

ASK THE EXPERT

products are available that contain sunscreen. Hair that has been bleached and/ or coloured is especially prone to sun damage.

SUN AND WIND

The major problems caused to the skin and hair by the wind are to do with its drying effects. The wind makes the ambient temperature seem lower (the chill factor), so that it is possible to be fooled into thinking that the sun is not as hot as it really is, and not use sufficient protection. When this is combined with the dry air of low humidity, the skin and hair can be damaged far more than necessary.

SWIMMING, THE SKIN AND THE HAIR

Risks to the skin and hair caused by swimming include:
- **In the sea:** exposure to UV radiation.
- **In a pool:** chlorine can irritate the skin and eyes, particularly in people who already have eczema.
- **Sea and pool:** salt and chlorinated water both dry and discolour the hair – chemicals in pool water bind to the hair, which can give

it a green/grey tinge, while minerals in salt water can turn hair a brassy colour, especially when combined with sun. Always rinse hair in fresh water before and after swimming.
- **Communal changing rooms** can increase the risks of picking up a verruca or athlete's foot infection.

BEAUTY AND THE BEACH

Temporary tattoos are currently fashionable on many beaches worldwide. Although described as henna tattoos, they usually contain other dyes such as PPD (P-phenylenediamine, also known as black henna) and kerosene. These are highly irritant to some skins, and set up irritant contact dermatitis at the site of the tattoo. Post-inflammatory hyperpigmentation may occur and the tattoo then becomes semi-permanent. Some children have been marked for years through having a black henna tattoo.

The story may not end there, because if you use a hair dye containing the same PPD chemical, you can develop a severe reaction in the scalp. The dye is also used in cheap sandals and can cause a rash on the feet.

Wind chill factor
A sea breeze can make temperatures feel deceptively cooler than they really are. Take care to stay in the shade and avoid the intensity of the midday sun.

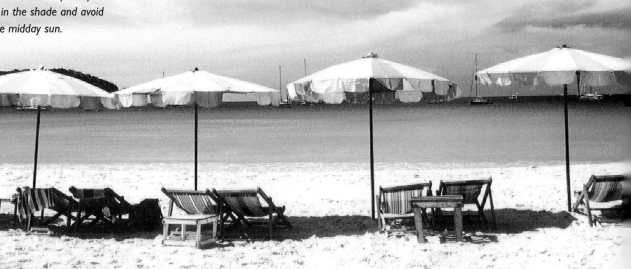

Winter and the skin, hair and nails

Winter is generally safer than summer for the skin, but winter sunlight can still be strong, especially when reflected by snow. Also, certain parts of the body can be affected by alternating extremes of cold and heat.

COVER UP FOR WINTER

Those who engage in skiing and other outdoor activities in snowy climates need proper protection from the cold, and also protection from increased exposure to UV radiation. For every 300m (1000ft) in height, UV exposure increases by 5 per cent. And snow reflects 80–90 per cent of UV light, compounding the problem. Layered clothing, consisting of several light, loose layers will trap warm air next to the body, yet provide adequate ventilation. Thermal underwear is a good choice for anyone who has to spend long periods outside in winter, topped by shirt, jumper, jacket and coat. The layered approach allows you to remove one or more layers indoors when it is warm.

A below-hip-length coat, made from a tightly woven fabric like corduroy, offers most protection from the cold. A coat with a hood and a warm lining is ideal.

Wear well-insulated gloves to prevent your fingers from freezing. Children (and adults) who play in the snow need waterproof gloves. In extreme conditions, consider wearing mittens over gloves.

Up to 40 per cent of total body heat escapes through the head, so it is important to keep it well covered. If you don't have a hood, use a hat, scarf and earmuffs for added protection. Insulated shoes or boots are a good idea, and in the snow, these must be waterproof. Warm pairs of socks should help to prevent chilblains; if wool socks feel too 'itchy' try wearing them over a fine cotton pair. Indoors in winter, the humidity is reduced because of central heating, so skin can become dry and itchy.

Red cheeks

A ruddy glow on the cheeks is not always a sign of good health. It is often associated with visibly dilated small blood vessels after long, continued exposure to the cold. It is more common in northerly regions, and is a reflection of the susceptibility of fair-skinned people to cold winds and chilly winters. Applying moisturiser – with sun protection – and vaseline to the cheeks can help.

Chilblains

Chilblains are itchy, burning red swellings which erupt after exposure to cold, but not necessarily freezing, temperatures. Children and the elderly are more commonly affected, but they can occur at any age.

Chilblains are caused by the constriction and expansion of blood vessels in the body's extremities in response to changing temperatures. They usually occur on the toes, heels, fingers, lower legs, nose and ears.

As there is no effective treatment for chilblains, it is best to try to prevent them: moisturise the feet, maintain good circulation and avoid cold exposure. The itching can be relieved with soothing products such as witch hazel or calamine lotion.

Protect against the elements
Wear well-insulated clothing that allows sweat to escape, but ensure adequate sealing around wrists, ankles and the neck, where body movement may allow cold air to enter.

SKIING AND SKIN SAFETY

General guidelines on protecting your skin apply while skiing and in other cold weather situations.

- Drink lots of water: the air in winter at altitude can be very dry so it's important to stay well hydrated.
- Don't drink alcohol or caffeine: alcohol opens blood vessels near the skin's surface, cooling the skin, and both are diuretics, increasing urine production.
- Dress in layers, avoiding cotton; wet cotton stays wet, breathable synthetics dry out.
- Take extra clothes for breaks: when you stop skiing you will need another layer.

- Take plenty of snacks to replenish lost energy: this will help to keep you warm and energised.
- Be weather wise: the weather in winter can change suddenly, leading to rapid body chilling. Remember that winter sun is reflected by snow; use skin and eye protection.
- Wear a hat.

Take cover
Dress warmly but don't forget to protect the skin that is exposed. UV intensity increases with altitude – there is less atmosphere to absorb the sun's rays – so use a high factor sunscreen at all times.

Heat and skin

Persistent exposure to a direct heat source can have a visible effect on the skin. Sitting in front of a fire means that the site of damage is commonly the front of the lower legs. The usual result is a brownish pigmentation in the affected area.

THE DANGERS OF FROSTBITE

Frostbite occurs when body tissues are frozen, which takes only a few seconds in extreme cold. The risk is increased in strong winds, at high altitude, or by touching cold metals. Older people and children are at greater risk than adults, as are those suffering from conditions which reduce the blood supply to the skin, such as diabetes and smoking.

Frostbite generally attacks exposed parts of the body which are at the extremities of the blood circulation, such as the toes, feet, fingers, ears, nose and cheeks. The condition can be deceptively pain-free, but the affected area appears waxy-white in colour until it has thawed. Depending on the length of exposure, deeper structures such as muscles, nerves, arteries and bone can be affected.

The extent of tissue damage is only appreciated on rewarming. With mild damage there is redness and pain, and the tissues return to normal in a few hours. More severe damage causes blistering, gangrene and permanent changes to nerve function, leading to increased sweating and impaired sensation.

Rewarming should be undertaken quickly, but gently. The best method is to place the sufferer in a water bath at 38°C (100°F), for no more than 20 minutes.

GIVING NATURE
A HELPING HAND

Most people attempt to improve on the skin and hair that nature has given them to some extent – using make-up and hair colorants is the norm rather than exceptional. However, more radical methods of modifying appearance are becoming increasingly common in our modern society.

 84

Changing the colour, texture and even length of hair has never been easier with growing numbers of products for home and salon use.

 88

The range of make-up products on the shelves is bewildering, but a few carefully selected items will be all that most people need.

 92

Painting finger and toenails can be a fun way to add a little flamboyance to your life, while extensions can disguise bitten or worn nails.

 94

Tattooing and body piercing are becoming increasingly popular, but serious thought is vital before a decision to proceed is made.

 95

Cosmetic surgery is not to be undertaken lightly. It is most successful when realistic outcomes are discussed with a reputable surgeon.

A daily makeup routine

There are no 'rules' about makeup: just please yourself. Many people find makeup enhances how they feel about themselves, and some say they feel 'naked' without it. But many others are happy not to use makeup on a daily basis.

If your life is a rush from the moment you get up, you might want to keep your daily makeup routine simple and quick, or dispense with one altogether. If you have the time and the personality, you might want to do more: iridescent face powder and glossy lips are too much for some first thing in the morning, but others wouldn't want to leave the house without them.

Now and again, before applying your makeup, have a good look in the mirror.

- Are you finding that your usual makeup is just not 'working' any more? It may be that your skincare routine could do with a change (your skin might have changed due to climate, age or hormones). Changing to a different moisturiser, for example, might make a difference (see page 53).

- Could your eyebrows do with a tidy-up? You could consider visiting a beautician for a proper shaping that you can then repeat. If you are going it alone, take it slowly and don't be overzealous. Remember that makeup works best when it is an enhancement of healthy skin, not a substitute for it.

THE SKIN OF THE FACE

Start by cleansing your skin and preparing it with a moisturiser and, if you feel you need it, a gel or cream around the eyes. Give your skin a few minutes to absorb this before proceeding, then create a base from a choice of products:

- **Tinted moisturiser** If you have dry skin, apply this on top of your first moisturiser, otherwise this can be used instead of a moisturiser. Tinted moisturiser is an excellent timesaver since it's a two in one product and gives a healthy look without covering the skin.

- **Liquid foundation** Apply this with your fingertips (the warmth of your skin will make it glide on more easily) or use latex wedges (readily and cheaply available, so you can throw them out after a few washes). Apply a few dots – you can always add more – to the centre of your face and work outward. You might feel that just covering any redness around the nose and the darkness under your eyes is enough.

- **Stick foundation** Apply to your face straight from the stick and work in with your fingers or a latex sponge.

- **Cream to powder foundation** Apply with the (normally included) sponge. This has quite a bit more coverage than the other products and is often referred to as a three in one product (foundation, concealer and powder).

Choosing colours

The best colour for foundation is a shade that matches your skin tone perfectly – the colour should almost disappear. If possible check this in natural light (take a mirror with you when shopping). For most people a yellow-toned foundation is the most flattering: pink-toned ones can make white skin look pasty and dark skin look grey. If you have dark skin look for golden tones to bring out the warmth in your complexion.

Working with nature
Often the most successful makeup is unobtrusive: face colours to match natural skin tone, well-shaped brows and lightly accented lashes can form a good foundation for a flamboyant choice of lip colour.

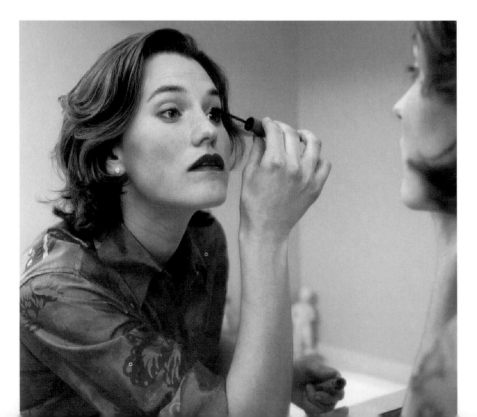

Hiding blemishes

Any blemishes and dark areas can be hidden with concealer. These are available as sticks (use a small brush for more accuracy) and liquid, which comes with its own brush in the bottle or tube.

Find one which is a shade lighter than your skin tone and one which is a match for it. A blemish is less noticeable with a matching covering, while under-eye circles vanish with a shade lighter. Try out brands with light reflective particles, they can be extremely effective.

Makeup artists are still divided over applying concealer before or after foundation: experiment to find out which works best for you.

Powder

One thing that makeup artists do agree on is that it is good to 'set' your makeup with powder, preferably loose powder applied with a puff. This is because loose particles – as opposed to compact powder which is applied with a flat sponge – 'lock' everything in place more easily. The colours that suit most people are yellow-toned or translucent powders. Stay away from the chalky pink ones. Any excess can be brushed away with a big powder brush.

On the other hand, if you're happy with a quick powder of your nose with your compact powder, stick to that if it suits you. You might, however, want to try loose to see if it makes any difference.

Blusher

If you decide to apply blusher, opt for the shade that most closely matches your natural flush. Apply it on the apple of your cheek: smile very widely and aim for the fleshy part, where your natural flush will appear.

Get a proper blusher brush if you use a powder blusher as the brushes supplied are too narrow and hard. If you use a cream blusher, which should be applied with your fingertips, apply it before the 'setting' powder.

EYE PRODUCTS

Eye products can have as little or as much impact as you want: you can keep your look minimal, go for glitter eye shadow and false eyelashes or anything in between.

Start with less of a product: it's always easier to add than it is to take away. Keep in mind that dark colours on the eyes make your skin seem to recede while light eye colours draw your skin forward.

Shadows

Your basic choices are cream eye shadow, powder eye shadow and loose eye shadow; all come in a variety of matte, shimmer, sparkle and gloss versions. Whatever you choose to experiment with, it is usually worthwhile getting some proper tools instead of using the ones supplied with the products; this often makes a product easier to apply and longer lasting.

Pencils and liners

Some people find hard pencils uncomfortable to apply. Liquid eyeliners (either a tube with brush or resembling a felt-tip pen) are best kept away from the inner rim of your eyes since they can cause

Baring all
Many women prefer the look of natural skin and do not use makeup regularly. Unadorned skin has natural colour.

irritation: stick to the area below the bottom lashes and above the upper ones. If you want to use eyeliner to define your eyes but find black a bit harsh for daytime use, you may find brown, brown-black or navy give a more satisfactory effect.

Eyelash curlers

For an open, awake look, an eyelash curler (metal, plastic or even heated versions) can work wonders. Makeup artists recommend a simple one that you squeeze over your lashes as close to your eyelid as is comfortable and hold in place for 5 to 10 seconds, repeating if necessary. Take care when removing. Only use curlers before applying mascara, otherwise you run the risk of breaking your lashes since they will stick to the curler when you use it.

Mascara

Mascara comes in many colours and varieties, including types that claim to thicken and lengthen the lashes. Whichever you choose, wipe the wand on the tube or with a tissue before applying so as not to overload the lashes. It's easier to apply a second coat than it is to get rid of any excess.

If you want the look of coloured lashes but are sensitive to mascara, don't have time to apply it daily, swim regularly or are a contact lens wearer who finds mascara irritating to the lens, you could consider having your eyelashes tinted: a tint should last 4–6 weeks.

Subtle difference
The best makeup enhances rather than disguises your natural skin: colours should be chosen to approximate your natural look.

LIPS

Some people find the sensation of wearing lipstick unpleasant. If you don't like lipstick but need something to prevent chapping, you could consider a clear lip salve or balm. If you do like lipstick, however, the possibilities are endless: lip-liner, lip-gloss, lip-glaze and of course lipstick, which is available not just in a stick, but also in tube and jar form.

Some days a bit of coloured gloss or dabbing a hint of lipstick on with your fingertips will be enough, but on other days you may want lip-liner, followed by lipstick and finished off with a high gloss. Whichever you choose, it's worth buying a decent lip brush for applying lipstick. This is especially important when you stray away from neutral tones. You will need a firm, small and flat brush to be able to apply the product accurately: it will also last longer when applied by brush.

Some experts suggest using lip-liner as the first step, others prefer outlining the mouth after the application of lip colour. Whichever you find works, remember you don't have to stick to your exact natural lip line. Play about and see what different effects you can achieve by adjusting an arch or a corner.

TRICKS OF THE TRADE

Invest in the best quality makeup and tools you can afford. Good-quality powder and lip brushes, for example, make products easier to apply and you will get a better finish: you'll also find it easier to experiment with styles and colours.

When it comes to selecting products themselves, personal preference, how important makeup is to you and your budget all play a part. You might, for example, be able to make your favourite, but fairly fast fading, cheaper foundation last a lot longer if you purchase a better quality setting powder.

Try out various brands and price ranges and do not be afraid to experiment. Have a look at products for different skin types – you may find you can swap the heavy day cream you've been using for a light moisturiser. Or a skin illuminating makeup base, which you can mix with your regular foundation, might be the answer for those days when you feel less is more.

Finally, if you find a product or shade you like, don't be discouraged from being loyal because somebody or some magazine tells you it's 'out' this season instead of 'in'. Makeup is all about what you like.

READING LABELS

Many people are allergic to some of the ingredients in day-to-day cosmetics, especially to lanolin used in foundations, powders, makeup removers and self tanners. Also known as wool alcohol, wool fat or wool wax, lanolin is produced by the oil glands of sheep. Chemically it is a wax rather than a fat and contains about 25 to 30 per cent water.

If you have been experiencing skin rashes, apply a little of a suspected product to an area of neck, upper arm or the bend of your arm, daily for about a week to see if it causes a reaction. If it does, check labels for wool alcohol and try to find products that do not contain it.

If you find problems with different products, see if there is an ingredient that pops up on a regular basis and avoid those products out for a time

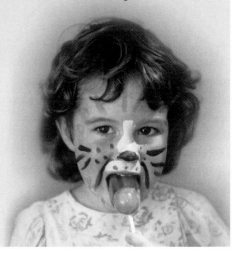

UNDER 8 YEARS
Face paints

Face paints are popular for parties and other special occasions, and most artists will use paints that are safe for children. It's legitimate to ask someone offering face painting in the shopping centre or at a fete what they are using and checking that's is intended for face painting – occasionally craft paints have been used. If you want to buy paints, look for toxic free and easily removable products; those suitable for small children are water based so that they wash off easily. Choose those that are labelled as non-staining, so that if any gets on clothes, it won't mark them. Most shops selling toys or party goods should be able to advise on suitable products.

to see if that makes a difference. If it doesn't, visit your GP. Your problem might, for example, be diet related, or you could be allergic to a substances you hadn't considered.

Skin-lightening products

Skin lighteners are used by many people, either to lighten skin overall or to even up patchy pigmentation. Of these those containing hydroquinone – which can damage the skin's genetic material – are banned in the EU. Azelaic acid and glycolic acids have caused skin irritation in some people.

CHILDREN AND MAKEUP

As with most things, the age at which children start experimenting with makeup is falling and in the last few years there has been a trend towards makeup for pre-teens – colour cosmetics, skin care and

fragrances for children who are still at primary school are now available in shops targeting this age group.

It can be difficult to regulate what pre-teens buy on shopping trips with friends, but parents have to decide where to draw the line. That doesn't mean that a four year old can't have fun with makeup, or that a twelve year old should be discouraged from a lick of moisturiser and a dab of lip gloss in the morning. You can, however, set some guidelines.

- Most schools ban makeup: support your child's school in this respect.
- Insist that makeup is scrupulously removed at bedtime.
- Discourage heavy makeup as a 'disguise' for spots: acne can be treated.
- Draw a distinction between trying out looks with friends at home, and what is appropriate, and when, outside the house.

POINTS TO CONSIDER

It is important to visit more than one surgeon. Deciding on the right plastic surgeon is crucial and you need to have seen at least two, preferably three, before making a choice – even if you end up going back to the first one you visited. This will add to the cost but it is a vital part of your pre-surgery research. There is no such thing as a free consultation; the charges will be added in to the surgery or treatment and a reputable surgeon will charge for your first consultation. At your consultation you need to:

- ☑ Consider the surgeon's qualifications and experience – always ask to see before and after pictures of surgeries performed.
- ☑ Ask about the complication rate.
- ☑ Ask about aftercare.
- ☑ Observe the staff: are they professional and organised? Do you like them?
- ☑ Consider the surgeon – do you like and trust him and do you relate well to him? Do you feel that he understands your needs and expectations?
- ☑ Ask the surgeon what he can do for you.
- ☑ Ask about costs and if there are any extras.
- ☑ Ask about which hospital he uses.

All of these factors, when considered together, will help you to rate each surgeon and to come up with an objective evaluation of their merits and whether they are right for you.

This indicates that the surgeon has had a basic surgical training. Surgeons who trained in the UK should be listed in the General Medical Council (GMC) specialist register; those who have been awarded the Certificate of Completion of Surgical Training (CCST) in plastic surgery will appear on the GMC specialist register for plastic surgery.

Qualifications are not a guarantee of excellence, but it is a good place to start. Your GP can recommend a reputable surgeon, but many people are reluctant to consult a GP about cosmetic concerns. Most reputable plastic surgeons belong to the British Association of Aesthetic Plastic Surgeons (BAAPS), so that is a good place to start (see page 160).

One factor that may set a reputable surgeon apart is a decision not to operate. Trained and experienced surgeons will refuse to operate when they believe that the requested surgery is not required or is inappropriate. They may refuse to operate if they have reason to believe that the request for surgery comes from someone other than the patient (for example, a boyfriend offering to pay for breast enlargement surgery). They are also trained to identify patients with a psychological disorder for whom surgery would not be the best treatment. Examples of this are people suffering with body dysmorphic disorder or those who are depressed and who believe that a facelift will find them their man or get them a new job. In these cases, the reputable surgeon may suggest a psychological assessment before surgery and may ultimately exercise the right to refuse to operate.

Seek counselling

Counselling is essential. You must discuss surgery with someone who can be objective. Your GP may be your first port of call or you may wish to discuss your ideas with a close friend or relative. There are professional beauty counsellors who will advise on the best surgeon for the procedure you want and who will provide information about the procedure and aftercare. Make sure that these counsellors are independent; they should charge for consultations. Beware of counsellors offering free consultations or those attached to cosmetic surgery clinics: they may be salespersons in disguise. Their bottom line is making money and they may not have your best interests at heart. *Never* consent to surgery without first having seen your surgeon on at least one, preferably two, occasions.

Know your budget

This is so important, and people frequently fall prey to dodgy deals because they use cost as the major determinant for their choice of surgeon and hospital. In a good cosmetic surgery practice, the patient coordinator or secretary will deal with money issues: the surgeon will not get involved. Get an idea of the costs involved when telephoning for an appointment. If the costs for a facelift are out of your range say so. The surgeon might be able to help you to achieve your objective by performing an eye-bag reduction or laser resurfacing while you save for the facelift. It is worth waiting an extra year to have surgery done by a qualified, experienced surgeon. Surgeons who are prepared to do deals will cut costs somewhere, and it will not be on their profits. The cost – not only financial – of repairing the damage done by an inexperienced or unqualified surgeon can far outweigh the cost of the surgery.

Be realistic about outcomes

Again this is difficult, and good surgeons will not operate if they feel that a patient's expectations are unrealistic and unachievable. There is no point in taking a photograph of Victoria Beckham to your surgeon and asking for lips like hers if you are a 50-something sun-worshipper who has smoked for years. A photograph of how you looked ten years ago, for example, will give something more realistic to aim towards.

Some surgeons use computer technology to 'morph' a digital picture of your face or body so that you can see how you will look after surgery. The technique can be helpful, but remember that surgery is not a precise science and the result might be different from what you were shown. Also beware of this technique if it is used as a sales exercise as the results cannot be guaranteed.

COMMON PROCEDURES

Non-surgical procedures include:
- injections of botulinum toxin;
- injections of 'fillers' such as collagen to plump out fine lines and wrinkles, raising them to the level of the surrounding skin;
- chemical peels (see page 124);
- dermabrasion and laser therapy for wrinkles, scars, tattoos or birthmarks (see pages 125–27).

Not all non-surgical procedures are exclusively in the domain of plastic surgeons: some dermatologists also undertake them.

BOTULINUM TOXINS

Injection of botulinum toxins is the most popular non-surgical cosmetic procedure in use today. It is becoming a 'lunchtime' procedure: it takes only minutes and involves no anaesthetic or sedative. The rapid increase in its use – 500 per cent in the last year – is mainly due to the fact that the Food and Drug Administration (FDA) in the United States has approved Botox® (Allergan Inc) for cosmetic use. Botox® is not the only botulinum toxin available, but its name has become synonymous with the treatment. Dysport® (Ipsen) and NeuroBloc® (Elan Pharma) are also available in the UK and the USA.

None of these products is licensed for cosmetic use in the UK (although this situation may change): these are prescription-only medicines and you need to be very careful whom you choose to administer them. Ideally, a qualified medical practitioner should give them, and at the very least, if they are to be given by a nurse, a doctor must have seen you prior to writing the prescription.

How do botulinum toxins work?

Botulinum toxins are given as injections into the muscles that underlie frowns, furrows and lines – mainly the frown lines, crow's feet around the eyes and horizontal forehead lines. Botulinum toxin is a neurotoxin that works by relaxing the muscles and by preventing them from contracting. Because the muscles are unable to contract the lines above them disappear. If the lines or furrows are very deep, it is sometimes necessary to 'fill' them with an injectable filler such as collagen after the botulinum toxin treatment has had time to take effect.

Botulinum toxins take two days to two weeks to reach their maximum effect. The injections need to be repeated after three to six months.

Side effects of botulinum toxins

It is possible to have an allergic reaction to the toxin when injected, although this is extremely rare and is probably due to the albumin solution in which it is suspended. After a period of repeated injections some people develop antibodies to the toxins which therefore become unable to achieve the desired effect.

Poor placement of the injections can lead to drooping of the features, particularly if the injections for

Non-surgical procedures are the most common cosmetic interventions performed by cosmetic surgeons and are most frequently performed on people under the age of 50.

forehead lines are given too far from the centre: this can cause the eyelids to droop. This is only temporary, but may nevertheless cause distress.

FACELIFTS

When most people think of cosmetic surgery, the image that comes to mind is of facelifts and of the taut, often overstretched look that seemed to typify the operation. The technical term for a facelift is rhytidectomy – literally, removal of lines. The operation appeals mainly to women from their mid to late 40s up to the late 60s but there is some evidence that women as young as 30 are considering this surgery and increasingly men are requesting it too.

Types of facelift

There are four basic types of facelift – if the surgeon you consult only does one type, consult someone else. All faces differ in the degree and extent of ageing, as well as in the sites of ageing: a good surgeon will recognise and advise the best technique for an individual face. There is no such thing as a formula facelift.

The most popular technique is the SMAS (submuscular aponeurotic system) lift in which excess skin is removed and the remaining skin is redraped optimally. It also includes tightening the SMAS layer (underlying muscles) and excess fat under the chin may be removed by liposuction.

Some surgeons may perform an extended SMAS lift, where the procedure is the same as for the SMAS lift except that more tension is placed on the layer of muscles, rather than on the skin.

The subperiosteal or MASK lift can be performed with an endoscope. The procedure involves freeing the

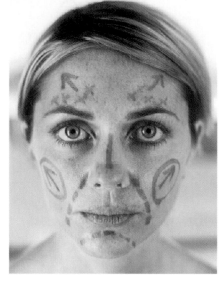

Facelift markers
Prior to surgery, sterile coloured marking pens are used to indicate incision lines and geographical reference points on the skin.

muscle from the bone so that it can be tightened and so that excess skin can be pulled up and excised.

The most extensive technique is a composite facelift which involves removing skin from the upper and lower eyelids, a brow lift and tightening of the face and neck muscles. Only very experienced surgeons are capable of performing this technique.

Getting the facts

While it is not necessary to know all the technical details, if you are considering a facelift you should know enough to be able to question your potential surgeon wisely. You should be aware that all facelifts involve making an incision at the temple (in the hairline) and that the different techniques create incisions – and hence scars – at other places, mainly around the ears.

A facelift is major surgery – as a minimum it will take three hours under a general anaesthetic. The recovery time, for those who obey the post-operative instructions to the

letter, is a minimum of two weeks before feeling comfortable in public again and it can be several months before all of the scarring and swelling finally settle down into the finished result. It is important to remember also that a facelift will not last forever. It will probably need repeating after about ten years.

EYELID SURGERY

Eyelid surgery (blepharoplasty) is performed on adults of all ages for two main reasons: to correct signs or effects of ageing, or to correct inherited traits. In the latter case, people may seek surgery as early as their 20s or 30s.

Reasons for seeking eyelid surgery

- Loose skin hanging down from the upper eyelids can obscure vision.
- Excess skin obscuring the natural fold of the upper eyelids.
- Droopiness of the lower eyelid showing white below the iris.
- Bags and dark circles with or without excess skin and fine creepy wrinkles of the lower eyelid.
- A puffy appearance of the upper eyelids – people may say your eyes look tired.

Eyelid surgery itself generally involves the removal of excess skin and fatty tissue from the upper or lower lids or both. The incisions can usually follow the natural contours of the eye and are well camouflaged when healed. Many surgeons are using a new approach, called a transconjunctival incision. This results in no visible scars at all as the incisions are made inside the eye.

Complications include the risk of haematoma formation – an accumulation of blood under the skin that may require removal. The eyes may also become dry, increasing the risk of infection. It usually takes at least two weeks for all bruising to subside and the result may take two or three months to become apparent.

Blepharoplasty is not the answer to all eye area problems: sagging eyebrows may be best treated by a brow or forehead lift, for example, and crow's feet may be smoothed by laser resurfacing or a chemical peel.

BREAST AUGMENTATION

Breast augmentation or enlargement is very popular, particularly in women who have completed their families and who would like to put some shape back into their breasts.

There are many types of implant available and your surgeon will discuss the most appropriate type for you. You need to be realistic when choosing your new size. Reputable surgeons will not increase a woman's bra size by more than two sizes at any one time. This is because the skin would have to stretch too much: this could be uncomfortable and increase the risk of capsule formation.

Breast implants are placed on top of, or underneath, the breast muscle, through an incision at the side of the breast. There will be a scar that may be visible when it has healed.

Following surgery under a general anaesthetic, you will be tightly bandaged for about a week. After this time, the surgeon will see you again to remove the stitches. You must wear a supportive bra (like a sports bra) for several weeks following the surgery, to ensure that the implants fix in the right place.

Complications of breast augmentation surgery are infection, haematoma formation and the formation of a capsule around the implant. This is a normal healing process, but sometimes it occurs excessively and the capsule may contract and compress the implant, causing the breast to feel harder than normal and perhaps distorting its shape. Occasionally implants need to be removed or exchanged because of these complications.

BREAST REDUCTION

Breast reduction surgery is sought by women who feel that their breasts are too large or whose breasts are so large they produce symptoms such as back and shoulder pain and also psychological distress. This is major surgery performed under a general anaesthetic, so you need to be fit and well before being considered for it.

The most common method of reducing the breasts involves three incisions. One incision is made around the areola. Another runs vertically from the bottom edge of the areola to the crease underneath the breast. The third incision follows the natural curve of the breast crease. After excess breast tissue, fat and skin have been removed, the nipple and areola are shifted to a higher position. The areola, which in large breasts has usually been stretched, is also reduced in size. Skin that was formerly located above the nipple is brought down and together to reshape the breast. Liposuction may be used to improve the contour under the arm. Usually, the nipples and areolas remain attached to underlying mounds of tissue, and this allows for the preservation of sensation. The ability to breastfeed may also be preserved, although this cannot be guaranteed.

Complications include bleeding, infection and poor healing. Occasionally the breasts appear uneven in shape or size, and sensation in the nipples is reduced or absent. Minor changes may be made at a later date if required.

LIPOSUCTION

Liposuction is the single most common cosmetic surgery procedure for both men and women. People seek it at all ages, usually for isolated pockets of fat in the buttocks, thighs, tummy, upper arms or chin. The best results are obtained when the skin has enough elasticity to spring back, so that a smooth and unwrinkled outline is achieved. Liposuction should not be used as a substitute for weight loss, and reputable surgeons recommend that patients are at their desired weight before undergoing the procedure.

Fat is removed by inserting a small hollow tube (a cannula) through one or more tiny incisions near the area to be suctioned. The cannula is attached by tubing to a vacuum pressure unit and guided by the surgeon; the suction device literally sucks away unwanted fat.

Following surgery the areas that have been treated will be bruised and there may be some swelling. The surgeon will apply tight pressure dressings or garments to help to produce a smooth even contour and these must be worn for as long as instructed. There may be some numbness in the treated areas, but feeling will return over two to three weeks, as the bruising and swelling subside.

The results of liposuction are permanent provided that your post-operative weight is maintained. If you do gain weight, it may be better distributed than previously.

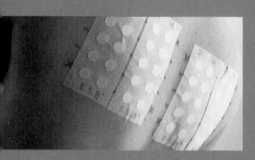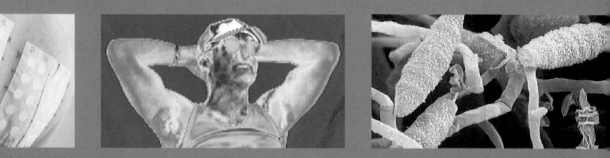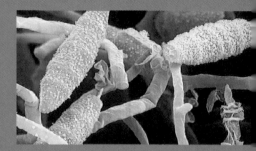

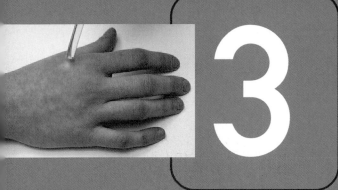

3

What happens
when things go wrong

Knowing what can go wrong

The skin's large surface area and complex make-up make it vulnerable to a wide variety of ailments, some inherited, some the result of infection, and some brought about by contact with the environment.

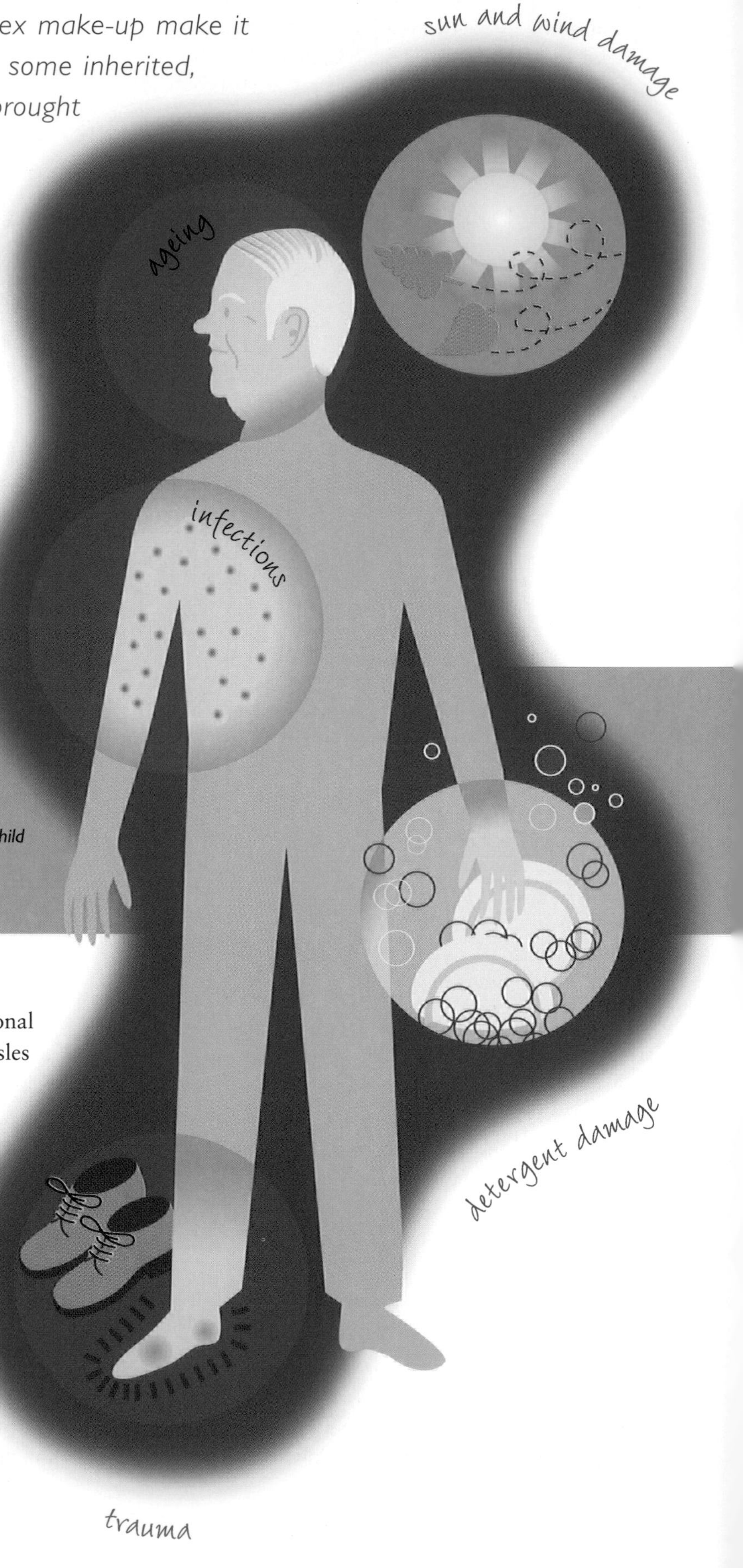

AGE-RELATED PROBLEMS

Some skin problems are more common at one age than at another. For example, a child is more vulnerable to infection, whereas an ageing adult bears the effects of many years' exposure to ultraviolet radiation.

Growing up

A baby's skin is more vulnerable than that of an adult, and therefore contact with the environment is the cause of most skin problems at this age. Infantile eczema, for example, is thought to be provoked by environmental

MORE COMMON

ACNE	ECZEMA
75,000 PER 100,000 (3 IN 4)	20,000 PER 100,000 (1 IN 5) CHILDREN
Three quarters of teenagers have acne at some point; the incidence is also increasing among adults with estimates suggesting that as many as 1 in 5 people aged 25 to 44 are affected.	This number falls to 1 in 12 adults; in the 1950s only 1 child in 20 was affected.

factors. Infections that affect the skin (caused by bacteria, viruses or fungi) are common. The traditional childhood illnesses chickenpox (see page 137), measles and German measles (rubella) produce skin rashes and are all caused by viruses. Because the immune system is less well-developed than it will later become, infections such as impetigo, a bacterial skin infection (see page 143), may persist or recur throughout childhood. Warts (see page 155) are another common skin infection, in this case caused by a virus.

Problems on all fronts

The skin faces daily assault from many sources, so skin problems are common. However, many are easy to avoid or treat.

sun and wind damage

ageing

infections

detergent damage

trauma

It is important to protect a child from too much ultraviolet radiation (UVR) from sunlight. This is because exposure to excessive amounts of UVR in childhood is thought to be a major cause of skin cancer in later life, especially if a child suffers sunburn: a single episode of blistering sunburn can be enough to trigger a cancerous growth.

Acne (see page 134) is the main skin problem worrying teenagers, and may persist into the 30s, and even beyond.

Getting older

As we age, the effect of UVR takes its toll, with creases, lines and wrinkles becoming common on areas of the skin exposed to sunlight. As damage from UVR accumulates, so does the risk of skin cancer. In addition, cigarette smoking promotes premature ageing of the skin that is especially noticeable on the face. Detergents such as washing up liquid will take their toll on the condition of hands and nails, unless protective gloves are worn.

What do liver spots have to do with the liver?

The answer is nothing, although they were once believed to be a sign of liver malfunction. A liver spot (also known as a sun spot or age spot) is called a lentigo by the experts (several are lentigines or lentigos). They are flat, harmless brown discolorations of the skin found on sun-exposed sites of the body such as the face, neck and backs of the hands. They are caused by long-term sun exposure, and can only be prevented by avoiding the sun before the age of 40. The new treatment for them is to use alpha- and beta-hydroxy acid gels and peels. A liver spot on the face may occasionally develop into a slow growing malignant melanoma, so if you notice a liver spot changing, seek a referral to a skin specialist.

ASK THE EXPERT

LESS COMMON

FUNGAL FOOT INFECTION	PSORIASIS	SKIN CANCER	LUPUS
15,000 PER 100,000 (1 IN 7)	3000 PER 100,000 (1 IN 33)	526 PER 100,000 (1 IN 190)	88 PER 100,000 (1 IN 1136)
At any one time, 15 per cent of the UK population has a fungal foot infection. Forty per cent of these also have a nail infection.	Most cases appear between the ages of 15 and 40.	Only 1 in 50 cancers are malignant melanomas; 75 per cent of non-melanomas are basal cell cancers, which have a cure rate of 90 per cent. Squamous cell cancer accounts for 20 per cent of cancers and has a cure rate of up to 80 per cent.	It is estimated that 50,000 people, mostly female, are affected by the autoimmune disorder lupus. It is more common in Asian and Afro-Caribbean women than in Caucasians, for reasons which are unclear.
	VITILIGO		
	1000 PER 100,000 (1 IN 100)		
	The incidence of vitiligo is fairly constant the world over.		

GENETIC INHERITANCE

Some skin disorders have a genetic cause. The common conditions eczema and psoriasis fall into this category, but it is thought in both these cases that environmental factors may also be involved. If there is a history of a severe inherited skin disorder in the family, a skin biopsy can be taken from a fetus, making prenatal diagnosis of rare conditions such as epidermolysis bullosa, ichthyosis (see page 143) and albinism (see page 135) possible.

GEOGRAPHIC AND RACIAL FACTORS

Skin diseases vary in frequency from one part of the world to another. This can often be because a particular infectious disease is more prevalent in a particular part of the world, as with leprosy (see page 145). In addition, the varying amount of pigment in the skin and the differing nature of the hair follicles in different racial groups make different racial groups more or less prone to certain problems with skin, nails and hair: skin cancer, for example, is far more common in Caucasians than in people of Afro-Caribbean origin..

CLIMATE AND THE WEATHER

Our skin protects us from the weather, but in the process it is inevitably changed, and not often for the better. These changes are mainly brought about by exposure to UVR – the sun is the biggest influence on the skin's health and appearance. Wind, rain and snow, however, can all influence the feel and look of the skin and hair, making skin too dry, rough or sore; lips are particularly prone to chapping in cold weather. Chilblains (see page 137) can develop on exposed hands and feet in very cold weather.

ECZEMA (DERMATITIS)

Eczema and dermatitis (see page 138) are often thought to be separate conditions, but as far as dermatologists are concerned the words are interchangeable. The primary defect in eczema is a breakdown in the barrier function of the skin, allowing antigens such as house dust mites and bacteria to penetrate the skin. This barrier defect may be inherited (atopic eczema often runs in families and is associated with asthma, hayfever and urticaria) or triggered by an allergic response to a particular substance, or by long-term exposure to some kind of irritant such as a detergent. Allergic contact dermatitis is most often set off by contact with nickel, but chemicals in glues, dyes, leathers, skin creams or cosmetics are all common causes.

SKIN TUMOURS

There are many cell types in the epidermis and dermis that can undergo changes from disease processes, and each cell type develops its own form of tumour. For example, basal cells in the epidermis can proliferate to produce harmless seborrhoeic warts or develop into malignant basal cell carcinomas. Melanocytes can produce harmless pigmented naevi (moles) or malignant melanomas that can be fatal if not picked up early (see page 130). The skin may also be the site of secondary spread of cancers that first developed in other parts of the body, such as the breast or the lymphatic system.

FUNGAL INFECTIONS

Skin-loving fungi called dermatophytes feed on keratin and give rise to various problems including athlete's foot (tinea pedis), toenail infections (onychomycosis),

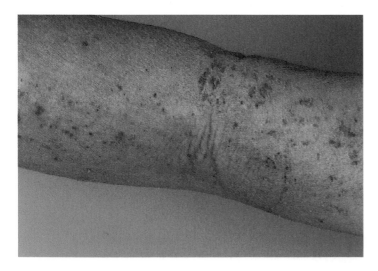

In the UK, 6000 new cases of malignant melanoma are diagnosed each year and 1700 people die from the disease.

ringworm of the body (tinea corporis), and scalp ringworm (tinea capitis). Fungi that affects humans can come from humans, animals or soil; the inflammatory response is most severe with fungi from soil, less severe with animal sources and milder when the source is human.

TRAUMA

The skin has amazing healing properties, and is able to restructure itself even after major injury. However, sometimes scar tissue does not stop forming but continues to grow at the site of injury. Excessive growth of connective tissue beyond the original trauma site is referred to as a keloid (see page 144). Keloids are most common on darker skins, and on the head and neck.

NUTRITIONAL DEFICIENCIES

A poor diet will often affect the skin. In regions where famine is common, the disease kwashiorkor caused by malnutrition leads to darker skin and the development of red-brown hair. Iron deficiency can make nails brittle and spoon-shaped, and may also cause hair to thin. There is an association between pernicious anaemia (an autoimmune disorder that prevents absorption of vitamin B_{12} in the stomach) and silver hair and blue eyes. (Premature greying of the hair is thought to be an independent autoimmune disorder.) Deficiencies of calcium can cause brittle nails, lack of copper can cause hair loss, and not enough fatty acids can lead to dry skin and hair. A deficiency of niacin may cause dermatitis, lack of vitamin B_6 can cause acne and hair loss, while anyone lacking in vitamin A could suffer from acne, dry hair and thicker, rougher skin.

HAIR LOSS

Hair loss can be caused by genetic factors (male pattern baldness); it can also result from drug treatment for some other illness (it is a common side effect of chemotherapy), from stress, or from a medical disorder (see page 141).

A typical case of eczema (dermatitis) on an arm
The inflamed itchy skin that characterises eczema/dermatitis affects one in five of all patients who attend a dermatology clinic. These patients may be any age.

Who's who – skin, hair and nail specialists

Experts in diseases and disorders of the skin, hair and nails tackle a wide range of problems, from the minor – removing a skin tag, for instance – to major life-threatening conditions such as skin cancer.

GENERAL PRACTITIONER

The family doctor is most people's first port of call with a problem to do with the skin, hair or nails. Many GPs have specific experience in dermatology, either from working in a hospital clinic under the supervision of a specialist dermatology team, or from extra study and gaining diploma qualifications.

PLASTIC SURGEON

A plastic surgeon is a doctor who first trained in general surgery, then undertook further training in plastic and reconstructive surgery. Plastic surgery aims to restore parts of the body that are deformed or damaged; the cause may be congenital, an injury of some kind, or the result of surgery for another problem.

ONCOLOGIST

An oncologist investigates and treats cancer. In cases of cancer of the skin, it is usual for an oncologist and a dermatologist to see the patient together in order to work out the best possible treatment. This may involve the use of drugs, surgery, radiotherapy, or a mixture of these.

OTHER HOSPITAL SPECIALISTS

All the following doctors are also hospital-based specialists, who in the course of their work become involved in the diagnosis and/or treatment of many different diseases and disorders of the skin.

- A **radiologist** uses imaging techniques such as X-rays, ultrasound, MRI and CT scanning to investigate various skin problems.
- A **radiotherapist** employs X-ray and radioactive substance therapies to treat cancers of the skin.
- An **immunologist**, based in the laboratory, investigates illness using techniques based on the workings of the body's immune system.
- An **immunotherapist** treats skin diseases, often skin cancer, with immune proteins to prevent the tumour cells growing and dividing.

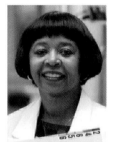

DERMATOLOGIST

This is a hospital-based doctor who has specialised in diagnosing and treating disorders of the skin, hair and nails. Most dermatologists have their own special subjects and research interests, and many have a great deal of experience in skin surgery and laser treatment. The majority have a lot of expertise in all dermatology problems as well as their own special interests. They work closely with oncologists, plastic surgeons and other medical specialists.

- A **histopathologist** is a laboratory-based pathologist who specialises in the analysis of body tissue samples.
- A **microbiologist** tests blood, urine, and body tissues for microorganisms that may be the cause of an abnormality in the skin, hair or nails.

TRICHOLOGIST

Trichologists are specialists in the diagnosis and treatment of hair disorders such as hair loss. They are generally non-medical experts (whose treatments have not always been subject to rigorous medical testing). Some dermatologists have a special interest in hair disorders.

CHIROPODIST/PODIATRIST

- A **chiropodist** treats foot and nail problems such as corns, bunions or ingrowing toenails; some have surgical experience. Patients with diabetes or other circulation problems need regular attention from a chiropodist.
- A **podiatrist** specialises more in disorders of foot function such as flat feet or overlapping toes and may supply shoe inserts to correct problems and to protect problem areas.

FINDING OUT WHAT IS WRONG

Because they are highly visible, skin problems can be among the easiest medical problems to diagnose. However, since several conditions produce similar-looking lesions, doctors can also call upon a battery of tests to identify the exact problem. These include blood tests, laboratory analysis of a sample of the rash, allergy testing, and the use of dyes to track the spread of a cancer.

Medical history and examination

Dermatology differs from other branches of medicine in that the problem is usually clearly visible. Keen eyes, a bright light and possibly a magnifying glass are often all that is necessary for a doctor to make a diagnosis.

WHAT THE DOCTOR LOOKS FOR

The doctor will want to know when the problem started, where on the skin of the body it originated, how it seemed to spread, and all details of any symptoms such as itching, pain, burning, blistering or fever. What seems to aggravate symptoms? Details of any methods the patient has found that alleviate symptoms are also very useful.

The doctor will ask the patient for a full description of any past skin problems, and their treatment, and will also want a general medical history, including details of all previous illnesses. Do any members of the patient's family have any skin troubles now (indicating the possibility of a transmissible infection) or have they had any in the past (indicating the condition might be inherited)?

The doctor will want a full list of any medications being taken by the patient. Many drugs can have an effect on the skin, either directly, as with an allergic reaction, or by altering the way the body reacts to sunlight. Details of the patient's diet are also asked for.

Information about the patient's job is important. What chemicals does the patient come into contact with? Do symptoms worsen at work? Hobbies must also be taken into account. Gardeners, for example, can develop an allergic rash brought about by contact with certain plants. Tropical fish can pass on a skin infection that would be very difficult for a doctor to diagnose without knowing that the patient keeps a fish tank. Has the patient been on holiday recently? Tropical worms, coral and sea urchins can all leave their marks on the skin.

THE EXAMINATION

To examine the skin properly, the lighting should be good. Most doctors prefer bright daylight. The doctor often needs to inspect the entire surface of the skin; it is always possible that some lesions may not have been noticed by the patient. If the face is affected, it helps the doctor if a patient does not wear makeup.

Describing changes in moles

Any pigmented mole, whether new or old, which shows three or more of the seven listed features, especially one of the first three, will be regarded suspiciously by a doctor, and will need to be removed and examined under a microscope.

- *Is an existing mole getting larger or starting to grow vertically? If a patient is over the age of 40 or so, is this a new mole growing?*

- *Does the mole have an irregular outline?*

- *Are there various shades of colour in the mole rather than it being all one colour? Any black coloration is particularly suspect.*

- *Is the mole greater than 1 cm in diameter?*

- *Is the mole inflamed or has it developed a reddish edge?*

- *Is the mole crusting, bleeding or oozing?*

- *Does the mole itch or hurt?*

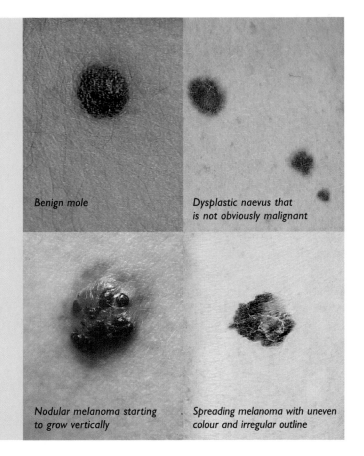

Benign mole

Dysplastic naevus that is not obviously malignant

Nodular melanoma starting to grow vertically

Spreading melanoma with uneven colour and irregular outline

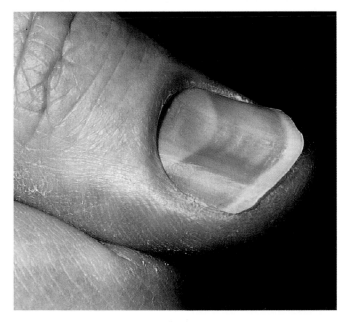

The nail condition koilonychia

The development of thin, brittle, concave, 'spoon-shaped' nails can occur as a result of anaemia due to iron deficiency. Why anaemia causes the nails to take on this shape is not known. If the anaemia is treated, the nails should return to their normal condition and shape.

THE SKIN AND NAILS AS BAROMETERS OF HEALTH IN GENERAL

There are a lot of diseases and disorders that affect the skin, hair or nails in addition to other organs in the body. A patient with a skin complaint of some kind may be surprised to learn, for example, that the problem is in fact diabetes, or a liver or respiratory disease.

Symptoms of the skin, hair and nails that indicate disease elsewhere in the body include:

- **Finger clubbing** This is a swelling of the soft tissues of the ends of the fingers, which makes the nails appear swollen and more rounded. It is a sign of lung and heart disease.

- **Liver palms** Redness of the palms may occur in pregnancy, but is usually associated with liver disorders.

- **Facial hair** Increased facial hair in women can be a pointer to an underlying hormonal imbalance such as that found in polycystic ovarian syndrome.

- **Koilonychia** This is a spooning and thinning of the nail plate, often associated with iron deficiency.

- **Beau's lines** These are horizontal lines that appear in the nails shortly after an illness such as a chest infection.

Tests and investigations

Although many skin problems are immediately obvious to the trained eye and easy to diagnose, some can be more difficult to identify accurately. General practitioners and hospital clinics can carry out an array of tests to help them to reach a diagnosis.

TESTS PERFORMED BY THE GP

After listening to a patient's story and carrying out a close physical examination, a family doctor may undertake further tests.

Blood tests

Sometimes a skin problem is an external sign of an internal illness such as liver disease or a cancerous tumour, or of a vitamin or mineral deficiency. For example, dry skin accompanied by hair loss might indicate an underactive thyroid gland; jaundice and spider naevi (red bumps with lines radiating out, resembling a spider's legs) may be symptoms of a liver disease. If a skin problem is suspected of being a symptom of something else, the first step in an investigation is for the GP to take a blood sample. Blood tests done in general practice would include tests for anaemia, kidney, liver and thyroid function, and tests to look for autoimmune diseases. Samples of blood are sent to the laboratory at the local hospital for analysis. The test results are returned to the GP, who may be able to treat the identified problem directly, or alternatively will refer the patient to a more specialist doctor.

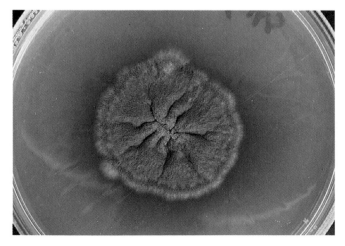

A fungus responsible for ringworm
A seven week growth of one of the fungi responsible for ringworm on the scalp (tinea capita). The fungus, Trichophyton violaceum, causes round scaly lesions that itch and give rise to patches of hair loss.

Investigation of infection

If the doctor suspects a skin condition is caused by infection, tiny samples of skin may be sent to a hospital laboratory to find out whether there are bacteria, viruses or fungi present. Samples are generally collected by rubbing a sterile swab, like a cotton bud, across the affected area. In the case of fungal infections such as ringworm (tinea), the doctor may take scrapings from affected skin, nail clippings, or a few hairs from the scalp.

Glass slide test

This is also called a diascopy. A glass slide or clear plastic spoon pressed onto the affected area of the skin causes the small blood vessels in the skin to constrict, so that the amount of blood within the skin is temporarily reduced, revealing whether redness in the skin is due to vessel dilation or bleeding into the skin, and allowing the true colour of a lesion to be revealed. Hopefully, this will aid in a correct diagnosis of the condition. Vasculitis (inflammation of blood vessels, see page 154), tuberculosis and meningococcal septicaemia are examples of conditions that prompt this type of test.

TESTS AT THE HOSPITAL CLINIC

When a family doctor is unable to make a diagnosis, the patient is referred to the dermatology clinic of the local hospital. Facilities there enable a wider variety of tests to be carried out.

SKIN BIOPSY

There are two main types of skin biopsy: punch biopsy and scalpel biopsy. Before either test, the area around the site of the biopsy is anaesthetised using a local anaesthetic injection such as lignocaine.
- A **punch biopsy** involves removing a 3–4mm wide cylinder of skin with a sharp instrument that bores a small hole into the skin. The sample is lifted free and

More than 18,000 skin biopsies are carried out each year in the UK.

Wood's light test

Wood's light is ultraviolet (UV) filtered through a nickel oxide prism. When Wood's light is shone on skin infected by certain fungi or bacteria, the skin becomes fluorescent.

a and **b** Scalp ringworm arising from fungi belonging to the Microsporum genus gives rise to blue-green fluorescence. Some other fungal skin conditions produce yellow fluorescence.

c and **d** The chronic bacterial infection erythrasma fluoresces coral pink – as shown here in a typical site between two toes.

In addition, areas of the skin where pigmentation is absent (see vitiligo, page 155) show up more clearly when bathed in Wood's light.

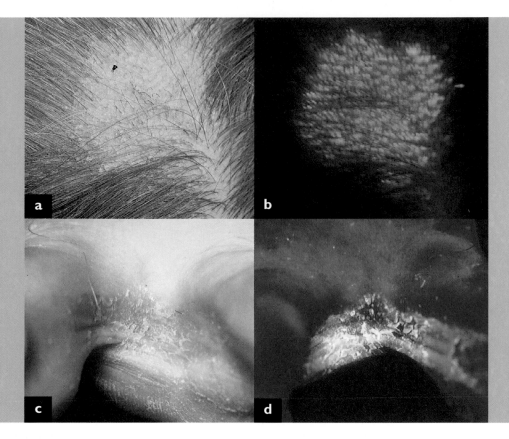

put into a bottle of preservative, then sent to a histopathologist for analysis. The cut on the skin is given a stitch or sealed with a diathermy needle.

• A scalpel biopsy is performed when a sample of tissue is required that is large enough to enable a comparison of normal and abnormal tissue. An ellipse of skin (shaped like an oval) that includes the area in question is removed, and the skin edges are then stitched together.

PHOTOGRAPHY

If there is concern that a mole is enlarging or changing, a digital photo may be taken in the clinic and filed with the patient's medical notes as a record of the mole's state at the time, to be compared with the appearance of the mole at the time of the patient's next check-up.

IMMUNOLOGICAL TESTS

Immunological tests examine the body's immune system, which helps to protect the body from harmful microorganisms, in order to investigate infections, allergies and irritants. They are very useful in the identification of skin ailments, and provide information that is often very valuable when it comes to deciding on the most appropriate treatment.

Skin prick tests

These try to identify which substance is triggering an immediate allergic response in a patient. They are also used to investigate the itchy red rash urticaria (see page 154). However, the results are not always helpful, as some patients show false positive or false negative results.

A patient must not take antihistamine medication for 48 hours before the test, because this will alter the test results. Single drops of commercially prepared dilute antigens are placed on the skin and the skin beneath each drop is pricked with a needle. The drops are then removed with a tissue, and ten minutes later the skin is examined for weals; any red, itchy patches or weals indicate a positive result. Skin prick tests are not performed if there is a risk of the patient experiencing a severe anaphylactic reaction.

Patch tests

These are used to establish whether a patient has contact dermatitis – that is, whether a rash is an allergic response brought about by contact with one or more substances. Drops from a standard selection of 'common culprit' allergens are placed on small aluminium discs set within a wide strip of adhesive tape. Discs and tape are then stuck

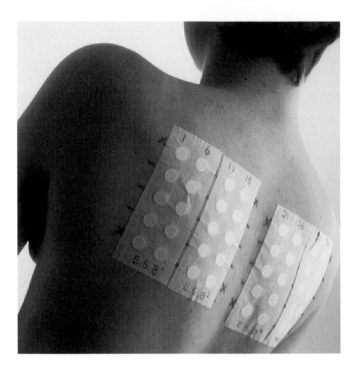

A patch test for contact dermatitis
*This young woman has four allergy test strips on her back.
On each test strip are ten discs, or 'patches', each of which tests for
skin sensitivity to a different allergen. If the skin underneath a patch
becomes inflamed, this indicates that the patient is allergic to the
substance under the patch.*

to the patient's back, so that the allergens come into
contact with the skin. If a particular chemical is suspected
that is not on the standard list, it will also be included.

The patches are left in place for 48 hours, then
removed after each site has been carefully marked.
Inspection at this time will show positive tests as being
red, swollen and even covered in blisters. The
skin is inspected again after 96 hours, to
see whether any further tests have come
up positive (these are late responses).
If any were positive at 48 hours
but negative at 96 hours, they
would be considered to be
irritant reactions.

If it is suspected that a rash
has been provoked by exposure
to ultraviolet (UV) light, more
specialised photopatch testing
may be available to check this
out. Two sets of the same allergens
are applied to the skin, as above.

Then, after the discs have been removed, one set of
allergens is exposed to a controlled dose of UV radiation.

Radioallergosorbent test (RAST)

A sample of the patient's blood is taken and sent to a
laboratory where it is tested for evidence of the patient
being allergic to certain foods or environmental allergens
such as the house dust mite. A RAST test is performed on
its own or together with a skin prick test, to see whether
they both produce the same results.

Immunofluorescence

This is a test used to differentiate between various types
of blistering diseases of the skin, such as bullous
pemphigoid, pemphigus (see page 150) and dermatitis
herpeteformis (see page 138). These disorders are caused
by the body reacting against its own tissues. Freshly cut
skin sections are treated with an antibody and labelled
with fluorescein, a dye which can be seen in UV light.
The sample is then examined using UV light, and the
location of the antibody on the cell membrane gives
diagnostic information about which particular skin
disease is present.

LYMPHOSCINTIGRAPHY

This is used primarily to investigate the cause of swelling
in the lower legs, to determine whether the cause is
blockages within the lymphatic channels or the veins,
but it can also be used to assess the spread of cancer such
as lymphomas affecting the skin (see mycosis fungoides,
page 148) and malignant melanoma (see page 147).
A radioactive dye is injected into a small lymphatic
vessel close to the surface of the foot, and then
a scanner is used to track the progress
of the dye up the leg and into the
lymph nodes in the groin, and
beyond if necessary.

Mycosis fungoides
*This transmission electron micrograph
image shows a slice through cancerous
white blood cells (lymphocytes) from
a patient with mycosis fungoides. This
condition primarily affects the lymphatic
system, but manifests itself as red scaly
patches on the skin that resemble those
caused by eczema and psoriasis.*

CURRENT TREATMENTS

The many treatments for diseases and disorders of the skin can be broadly divided into two categories: those designed to treat large areas and those that enable pinpoint accuracy in order to remove tiny growths and other lesions without damaging the skin around them. Creams and lotions can cover extensive areas, as can phototherapy. When skin has been badly damaged, skin grafting is sometimes required. Doctors freeze, scrape, shave or burn off many types of benign growths and markings – or even vaporise them with a laser. For life-threatening malignant melanomas, however, the preferred option is still to cut out the tumour and surrounding tissue with a scalpel.

Light treatments

Specialists use laser light and ultraviolet light therapies – alone or in combination with drugs – to treat a variety of skin ailments, from chronic conditions such as psoriasis to cancers of the skin.

TOPICAL PHOTODYNAMIC THERAPY (PDT)
Topical photodynamic therapy is used to treat a variety of premalignant skin lesions and is currently being tested in the treatment of some malignant tumours. First, a cream that contains a light-sensitive drug is spread onto the area of skin to be treated. A few hours later, a light (generally laser light) is shone onto this area; the light is set at a particular wavelength that will react with the photosensitising drug in the cream. Together, the light and the drug work to destroy the unwanted cells.

This technique is useful for treating areas of skin that have a number of lesions that need removing, as can be the case with premalignant skin conditions such as actinic (solar) keratoses (see page 134) and Bowen's disease (page 137).

A new development in topical PDT
The Paterson lamp is a new and potentially more convenient alternative to laser light when carrying out topical photodynamic therapy. The lamp uses lenses and fibre optics to produce an intense light from an electric current.

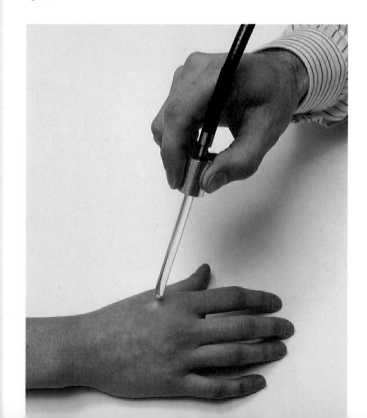

Photodynamic therapy is not yet as widely available as it might be, and does not have the back-up data on long-term effectiveness enjoyed by other treatments. But PDT is a particularly useful way of treating areas of skin that might heal poorly after other treatments, such as skin on the lower legs. Other advantages are minimal scarring and a reduced risk of infection compared with other treatments.

ULTRAVIOLET PHOTOTHERAPY

Many patients with inflammatory skin disorders observe that their skin improves significantly if they spend time outdoors exposed to the ultraviolet radiation (UVR) in natural sunlight. With the therapeutic benefits of UVR in mind, treatments have been devised that provide patients with an artificial source of UVR, thereby improving their skin conditions. These treatments are carried out within a controlled hospital setting.

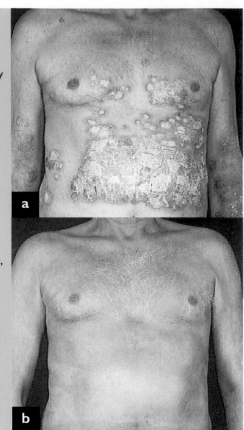

PUVA therapy for psoriasis

a One of the conditions for which ultraviolet phototherapy is particularly effective is psoriasis. This skin condition is characterised by a rapid turnover of skin cells, resulting in red patches covered with silvery scales. Ultraviolet phototherapy comes into play when the psoriasis has become resistant to drugs applied topically as creams, or there is a large area of skin requiring treatment.

b After six weeks of PUVA sessions, the skin has cleared up dramatically. However, PUVA treatment cannot be continued at this level indefinitely because of the risk of premature skin ageing and of skin cancer. Therefore, since the underlying causes of the disorder remain, it is likely that the psoriasis will return at a future date.

UVB phototherapy

Regular exposure to artificial UVB light rays administered by a lamp can be a very effective way of managing a number of diseases of the skin, particularly psoriasis. Careful monitoring is vital as UVB tans the skin and too much can burn it; also, as with sunlight, excessive exposure can cause the skin to prematurely age and increase the chances of developing a skin cancer. A factor in deciding whether or not to choose UVB phototherapy is whether the patient is fair skinned and therefore burns easily. Typically, UVB therapy is first given three times a week for six weeks, and then the patient's condition is reviewed, and a 'maintenance programme' is devised.

PUVA therapy

A more potent form of light treatment is PUVA. This combines taking a drug, psoralen, and UVA phototherapy. (P plus UVA forms the acronym PUVA.) The drug is usually taken by mouth, although it is sometimes applied in the form of a lotion to allow small areas of the body to be treated specifically. Two hours later the skin is exposed to UVA radiation from a fluorescent lamp. The UVA light enhances the effect of the drug on cells in the skin.

There is no doubt that PUVA therapy is a very effective treatment for psoriasis in particular; also for eczema and other less common skin conditions. It can be used to treat mycosis fungoides, a low-grade cancer of the immune system that affects the skin (see page 148). Treatment is generally required twice weekly for six weeks or so.

As with any treatment involving exposure to UVR, PUVA can produce a sunburn-like reaction. Patients taking psoralen in tablet form find the skin becomes very sensitive to light in the hours after a treatment session. So they have to cover up from the sun, and wear sunglasses. There is also a risk of skin cancer, particularly for patients who need repeat treatments of PUVA over a long period of time. (Due to the risk of carcinoma of the penis, male genitalia should be covered during treatment.) As a result of this cancer risk, PUVA treatment is carefully monitored and tends to be prescribed only after UVB phototherapy has been found to be ineffective for some reason.

Drugs for skin problems

There are a number of topical and systemic treatments for acne, eczema and psoriasis – the prevalent skin problems in society today – as well as treatments to solve or soothe a range of bacterial, viral and fungal infections, sunburn, and the effects on the skin of chemotherapy.

Drugs can be administered topically (locally) directly to the part of the body requiring treatment or systemically, that is in such a way that the body as a whole is affected (as with tablets and medicines taken by mouth, for instance). Topical drugs designed to treat the skin consist of a 'vehicle', also called a base, in which there is usually some kind of active ingredient. Vehicles include the following: lotions, thicker 'shake lotions' such as calamine, creams, gels, ointments, and pastes. Vehicles hydrate the skin, and they can have an anti-inflammatory effect and help the active drug to penetrate the skin.

The advantage of topical drug treatment is that the drug is delivered directly to the skin with minimal risk of side effects affecting the body as a whole. However, to be truly effective the drug must be able to penetrate the skin's outermost layers and its ability to do this is influenced by a variety of factors:
• the drug itself and its concentration;
• the age and existing degree of hydration of the skin;
• the type of vehicle.

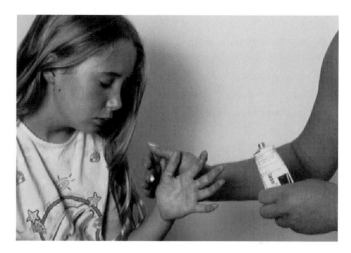

A soothing cream for itchy skin
Emollients are an important part of the treatment of many skin conditions. Regular applications of an emollient to the problem area – in this case an itchy blistering rash caused by contact dermatitis – help to keep the skin soothed, smoothed, flexible and hydrated.

If a topical preparation is used correctly for an appropriate period of time but does not produce the desired effect, a doctor may at this point consider prescribing systemic therapy.

PSORIASIS

Psoriasis (see page 151) is characterised by patches of flaking skin. Treatment aims to relieve inflammation and scaling, and to reduce the area of skin involved. The choice of treatment depends on which part of the body is affected, how much skin is affected, and how well the condition and its various treatments are tolerated. Topical therapy is the mainstay for mild to moderate psoriasis, while systemic or other specialist treatments are prescribed in severe cases.

Topical therapies for psoriasis
• Calcipotriol and tacalcitol are synthetic vitamin D preparations that block abnormal division of skin cells, increase cell maturation and modify the immune response that causes inflammation. For many doctors they are the first-choice topical treatment for psoriasis.

Dovobet: a breakthrough in the treatment of psoriasis

Dovobet is a new topical drug treatment for psoriasis sufferers that is the most significant advance in the treatment of this condition in the last decade. It combines two active ingredients already being used separately to treat psoriasis: calcipotriol and betamethasone. Calcipotriol is a derivative of vitamin D that slows down the excessive production of skin cells which characterises psoriasis. Betamethasone is a corticosteroid that reduces inflammation. Dovobet comes in the form of an ointment and is applied twice daily for up to four weeks. The improvement in the patient's condition is generally fast and dramatic, often removing the need for phototherapy or systemic drug therapy.

- **An emollient** may be all that is needed in mild cases.
- **Coal tar preparations** are available as creams, pastes and bath additives and may be used up to three times a day. However, they can smell unpleasant and be messy to use. Tar products can also stain skin temporarily and clothes and bedding permanently.
- **Salicylic acid** is often mixed with other ingredients, such as coal tar and dithranol, to make up a topical preparation. It loosens and removes thick scaly patches.
- **Tazarotene** is a derivative of vitamin A. It can be used to treat mild to moderate psoriasis, where up to a tenth of the body surface area is affected. It irritates the skin a lot, which limits its usefulness. Women who may become pregnant must use adequate contraception during treatment, because tazarotene can cause deformities in fetuses.
- **Dithranol** is an effective topical preparation for psoriasis but must be used carefully because it can severely irritate the skin, and permanently stains clothing, bedding and so forth. The drug is initially used at a low strength with the concentration being slowly increased during a course of treatment. It is applied as a cream, ointment or paste to affected skin only, then removed after an hour or less. Dithranol slows down the rapid rate of cell division that causes skin thickening. It is often combined with coal tar or salicylic acid.
- **Topical corticosteroids** (often just called steroids) may be used in difficult cases for short periods only. They can help with skinfold areas and to counter irritation caused by dithranol.

Systemic drugs for psoriasis
A small number of people do not respond to topical treatment or relapse very quickly afterwards. Systemic treatment under specialist supervision may include the use of the vitamin A derivative acitretin, the anticancer drug methotrexate, or the immunosuppressant cyclosporin.

ECZEMA
Most people with atopic (hereditary) dermatitis or eczema are treated with topical therapies.

Topical therapies for eczema
Topical therapies for eczema have three aims: healing the skin; preventing flare-ups; and treating any symptoms.

Psoriasis affects 1.5 million people in the UK and 7 million in the United States.

- **Emollients and moisturisers** smooth the surface of dry skin and help the skin to retain its moisture and become soft, smooth and flexible. When used correctly they can allow a lower dose of corticosteroid to be used without reducing its effect. Available as lotions, creams, ointments, soap substitutes and bath oils, they need to be used frequently to be effective.
- **Topical corticosterids** are used to control flare-ups of exzema. They inhibit the production and action of chemicals that cause inflammation in the skin, thereby reducing inflammation and itching. The steroid must be of a suitable potency for the area to be treated, and it must be applied sparingly, with use limited to the shortest time needed for a clinically acceptable effect. Skin thinning and stretch marks can occur with chronic use, and hypersensitivity to ingredients may lead to symptoms becoming worse.

Systemic drugs for eczema
- **Oral corticosteroids** are occasionally prescribed to quickly control a severe flare-up of eczema. They are usually taken at high initial doses, which are then reduced every few days over a course of 3–4 weeks. As the dose is reduced, topical steroids are increasingly used to counteract the disease flare-up that can occur on withdrawal of the oral steroids. Patients on systemic steroids must carry a steroid card.
- **Antibiotics** may be used when eczema is infected. The most commonly implicated organism is Staphylococcus aureus (staph), which can be treated with oral antibiotics for 7–10 days. Flucloxacillin is effective in 90 per cent of staph infections. Erythromycin is useful for penicillin-allergic people. Recurrent infections can be treated with antiseptic bath oils such as Oilatum Plus, and emollients such as Dermol 500. Topical antibiotics such as fusidic acid should be used only under supervision; short courses cause no problems but prolonged use can lead to drug resistance.
- **Antihistamines** of the older, sedating type may help at night-time for their sedative properties if itching is preventing sleep. Because the itch of eczema is not caused by histamine release, non-sedating antihistamines should not be used.
- **Evening Primrose oil** (gamma linoleic acid) is a controversial treatment with conflicting evidence about

How corticosteroids affect inflamed skin

a Skin becomes inflamed when irritation of skin by allergens and other irritants provokes the release of inflammatory mediators (chemicals that cause inflammation) from white blood cells. These chemicals cause blood vessels close to the skin's surface to dilate, making skin hot, swollen and red.

b Corticosteroids (also called steroids) are applied to the inflamed skin and absorbed, resulting in inhibition of the inflammatory mediators. Blood vessels return to normal and as a result the swelling, redness and heat of the skin is reduced.

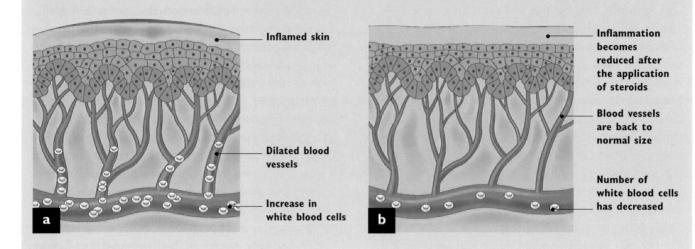

a — Inflamed skin — Dilated blood vessels — Increase in white blood cells

b — Inflammation becomes reduced after the application of steroids — Blood vessels are back to normal size — Number of white blood cells has decreased

its efficacy. For patients with very dry skin it can be a very effective way of reducing dryness, and of reducing inflammation in the skin.

TREATING ACNE

Response to treatment is relatively slow and patients need to realise that it may take up to six months before they see a significant improvement in their condition. But it is very important that a patient carefully maintains the prescribed treatment regime: poor compliance can lead to bacterial resistance and significantly reduce the effectiveness of the treatment.

Topical therapies for acne

Topical therapies remain the mainstay for the treatment of mild acne. They include drugs that influence the growth and function of acne bacteria and inflammation – known as comedone formation.

- **Benzoyl peroxide** has antibacterial properties. While benzoyl peroxide treats inflamed and non-inflamed skin effectively, it can cause irritation and bleaching.
- **Topical antibiotics** are helpful in reducing inflammatory acne lesions like papules (small raised bumps) and pustules. Clindamycin and erythromycin are common

choices. Topical tetracycline is also used but can leave a residue on the skin that fluoresces under ultraviolet (UV) light.

- **Topical retinoids** (adapalene, isotretinoin, tretinoin) are anti-comedonal therapies that are most effective in reducing blackheads and whiteheads. A common side effect is skin irritation. Alternating use of topical antibiotics and topical retinoids can produce good results. Patients using topical retinoids should avoid excessive UV light.
- **Topical combination preparations** include antibiotics and anti-inflammatory agents such as erythromycin plus benzoyl peroxide or zinc. These combination preparations appear to induce less bacterial resistance than the use of topical antibiotics alone.

Systemic drugs for acne

Oral therapies for acne can be divided into three groups: antibiotics, hormonal therapies and retinoids (the best known of which is isotretinoin).

- **Antibiotics** taken orally have been the mainstay of treatment for inflammatory acne for years. They are anti-inflammatory and reduce the activity of acne bacteria. Studies have shown that minocycline is the

How medication can affect skin and hair

The skin can react adversely to medications for many different kinds of ailments. Itching and rashes are the most common symptoms. In addition, hair loss may be triggered by reactions to drugs taken to fight a variety of diseases and disorders.

WHEN DRUGS CAUSE A SKIN PROBLEM

Reactions by the skin to medication may be caused by several different mechanisms; in many cases the exact mechanism is unknown. Hypersensitivity reactions are the most common causes of drug rashes. Other causes are photosensitivity, accumulation of the drug in the skin, or exacerbation of a pre-existing skin condition.

Symptoms of skin hypersensitivity reactions include itches and rashes, also wheezing and anaphylaxis (shock-like symptoms brought on by a sudden histamine release). Drugs responsible include: aspirin, antibiotics (especially penicillins, cephalosporins, sulphonamides), anti-epileptics, allopurinol and gold. Most rashes clear a week or so after the patient stops taking the drug that is the cause.

Drugs that cause photosensitivity rashes triggered by sunlight include: antibacterials such as tetracyclines and sulphonamides; diuretics such as thiazides; drugs for irregular heart beats such as amiodarone; and anti-psychotics like phenothiazines. Patients on these medicines are likely to need a high-SPF product for extra protection before going out into the sun.

WHEN DRUGS CAN CAUSE HAIR LOSS

Chemotherapy drugs damage normal cells as well as cancer cells. Healthy cells that are affected often include those in hair follicles, sometimes resulting in temporary hair loss. If hair loss occurs, it usually starts within a few weeks of starting treatment. The amount of hair lost depends on the combination of drugs taken, the dose and the way the individual's body reacts to the drugs. Loss of hair from the scalp may be partial or complete: eyebrows, eyelashes, body and pubic hair may also be lost.

With some chemotherapy drugs, wearing a specially designed 'cold cap' before, during and after each treatment session prevents hair loss by temporarily reducing the flow of blood to the scalp and thereby the amount of anticancer drug that reaches the hair follicles, and by slowing the metabolism of the follicles, making them less susceptible to damage. A number of other drugs can cause hair loss including anti-thyroid drugs, anticoagulants and certain combination contraceptive pills.

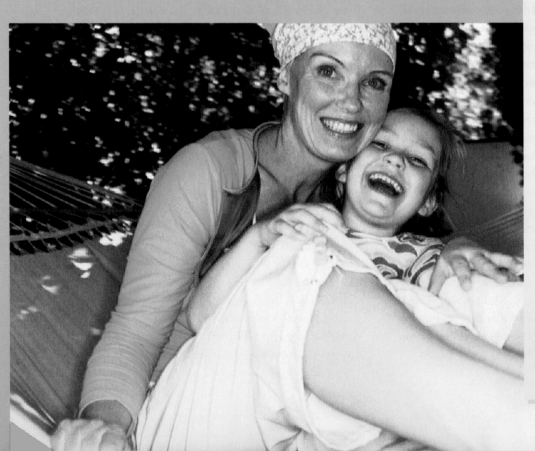

Tips for hair while undergoing chemotherapy

- If the chemotherapy is likely to cause hair loss, get hair cut short before treatment begins and use gentle hair products.
- Try not to comb or brush the hair too roughly – use a soft brush.
- Do not perm hair during chemotherapy or for 12 weeks after treatment.
- Only use mild vegetable based colorants – check with a hairdresser or chemotherapy nurse.
- Do not use heated styling products, including hairdryers.

If severe hair loss does occur, a patient who feels self-conscious about it could try wearing a scarf or hat when going out, or ask the chemo nurse or doctor about a wig.

Basic surgical treatments

There are a host of ways to remove unwanted or potentially harmful growths from the surface of the skin. Treatments range from cutting to freezing to burning, with bleeding stopped at source by cauterisation.

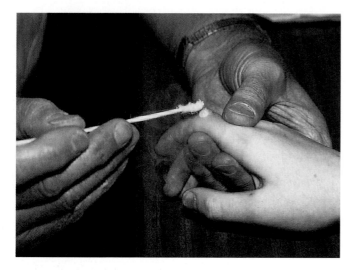

Cryotherapy to remove a wart
A wart on a finger is being treated with liquid nitrogen on a cotton bud. The liquid nitrogen freezes the wart solid. As the wart thaws a blister forms, and the wart is shed with the resulting scab.

CRYOTHERAPY

The use of cold to kill tissue is known as cryotherapy, or cryosurgery. This is a widely used treatment for a range of dermatological problems. It involves the application of a freezing agent to the affected skin, which causes damaged cells to burst and die, due to the rapid freezing and then thawing that takes place.

The most common freezing agent used today is liquid nitrogen. The liquid nitrogen is applied for between 10 and 20 seconds to the site of the lesion, using either a spray gun from a distance of about 10mm (½ inch), or a cotton wool swab.

Typical conditions that can be treated in this way include warts and verrucas, freckles, liver spots on the back of hands, and some skin pre-cancers and cancers.

Cryotherapy can be quite painful, and will cause inflammation and in some cases blistering. Sometimes a mild painkiller is needed to relieve discomfort caused by swollen and inflamed skin. Occasionally, cryotherapy can cause mild scarring or a permanent change in colour of the treated skin, especially in dark-skinned patients.

CURETTAGE

Another technique which allows the removal of simple skin lesions is curettage. A local anaesthetic having been injected into the skin, the skin lesion is scraped off with a sharp-edged curette spoon. The base of the skin, now raw and oozing or bleeding, is sealed by cauterisation.

Curettage is only possible if the material being scraped off is more frail than the surrounding skin, or when there is a natural cleavage plane between the lesion and the normal tissue that surrounds it. The resulting shallow wound heals by a combination of wound shrinkage and skin rejuvenation.

Using this method, a number of lesions can be treated in a relatively short period of time. The final cosmetic results can be excellent and there is very little post-operative discomfort. The disadvantage of curettage as a technique is that because the lesion is simply being

> ## " EXPERIENCING CURETTAGE
>
> *A small nodule developed on the side of one of my toes, which bled easily and frequently. My doctor referred me to the local dermatology clinic to have it looked at.*
>
> *The dermatologist told me that it was nothing to worry about: it was a pyogenic granuloma, which can appear after skin has been cut or damaged in some way. He sent me to another doctor in the clinic to have it removed.*
>
> *First, the doctor cleaned the area around the granuloma, then she injected a local anaesthetic between two toes. After the anaesthetic had taken effect, she scooped out the growth with a tiny curette spoon and then she applied an electrically heated wire to the cut skin to seal the tiny wound and prevent any bleeding. And that was it. The procedure was painless throughout and took about ten minutes, most of which time was spend waiting for the local anaesthetic to work.* "

scraped off the top layer of skin, there is always a small but recognisable risk that the lesion may recur.

ELECTROCAUTERY

Electrocautery is a very neat way of stopping any bleeding on the skin's surface. A wire is heated sufficiently by electrical conduction to produce enough heat to burn and thereby destroy the cut blood vessels and so put an end to bleeding from an incision in the skin. This technique is also used to burn away warts and other growths on the surface of the skin.

ELECTROSURGERY

Electrosurgery involves the use of an electric current to cut or burn tissue in a controlled manner. It is most frequently used to cut away lesions of various kinds. There are different methods suitable for different conditions and situations.

- **Cutting diathermy** is a technique that uses an electric knife – a diathermy knife, actually an electrode – to cut tissues. There is very little bleeding from capillaries because the cut edges are immediately cauterised. Sometimes a diathermy snare or needle is used instead.
- **Electrofulguration** destroys tissue with sparks sprayed from an electrode that is not actually touching the lesion, thus keeping destruction and scarring to a minimum. It is used to remove small skin growths such as nodules and warts.

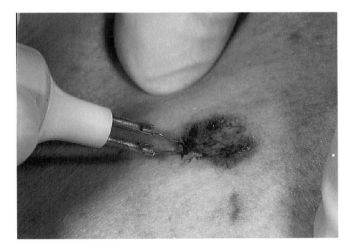

Electrocautery on the back of a hand

Electrocautery is taking place here in order to clean, seal and tidy a wound after a shave excision. A shave excision is used for the removal of benign growths such as skin tags. The growth is shaved off the skin with minimal disturbance to the skin below it.

- **Electrodesiccation** involves touching a lesion with an electrode, causing slightly deeper tissue destruction. It is often followed by curretage. This method can remove a wide variety of small growths. One use is the treatment of eyelid xanthelasma (see page 155) by removing these little fatty deposits that can develop around the eyes.
- **Electrolysis** is employed to remove unwanted terminal hairs. A needle having been passed into the hair follicle, an electric current is used to destroy the hair root.

SKIN EXCISION

When removing a mole or other growth from the surface of the skin by means of surgical excision, the same procedure is followed as for a scalpel biopsy (see page 108). The surgeon begins by drawing an ellipse on the skin's surface around the area to be removed. The ellipse is generally about three times as long as it is wide. The skin is cleaned and local anaesthetic is administered. The surgeon uses a scalpel to cut along the two curved lines that make up the ellipse, as far down as the layer of subcutaneous fat. The growth and the skin surrounding it are removed and the two cut surfaces are stitched together; generally only a few stitches are needed.

SURGICAL REMOVAL OF SKIN TAGS

Snip excision is a simple technique for the removal of small skin tags. The stalk of the skin tag is held away from the skin and snipped off at its base by a pair of sharp scissors. This often results in the spontaneous arrest of any bleeding. There is usually no need for a local anaesthetic unless a larger skin tag requires bleeding to be stopped with a stitch or cauterisation.

REMOVING A LIPOMA

A lipoma is a benign tumour made up of fat cells; it shows up as a lump below the skin. If it is unsightly or causing discomfort, it can be removed by means of a simple excision of the fat through a cut created in the overlying skin. The only disadvantage of this procedure is that there is the potential to produce a rather large scar. To keep the incision (and resulting scar) to a minimum, the lipoma may be broken up into smaller pieces before being brought out through the incision made in the skin. Alternatively, the fat within the lipoma can be fragmented and removed by the procedure known as liposuction (see page 99).

Skin grafts and transplants

Skin grafting involves taking healthy skin from one part of the body and placing it over a damaged area of skin instead. A graft allows injured skin to heal more quickly and effectively, and with less scarring, than would otherwise be the case.

WHEN IS A SKIN GRAFT NEEDED?

A skin graft is required when a defect in the skin is so large that it is not amenable to natural healing or closure with stitches. Such a defect has usually been caused by a burn or other injury, or by surgery (to remove a skin lesion, for example). One treatment option is that a flap of skin is brought over from a neighbouring area and grafted onto the defect. Alternatively, skin from a site elsewhere is transplanted to the damaged area – this is a straightforward skin graft.

MAKING A FLAP

A flap is a patch of skin that has been mostly cut away from the body but left attached at one end so that its blood and nerve supply is retained. The free end of the flap is stitched into the area to be repaired and when the flap has healed in place (a process that takes two to three weeks) the flap is cut free from its source and fully sewn in.

- A **local flap** uses skin that lies right next to the area to be covered. Sometimes the adjacent skin is stretched before it is used as a flap; this is done by inserting a balloon-like device under the skin beside the area to be covered and then slowly allowing the balloon to expand. This process is called tissue expansion. Because the skin of a local flap already has an intact blood supply, and is so similar to the skin that has been removed, the final result is often far superior to a more traditional skin graft, and there is a much smaller chance of the new skin failing to 'take'.
- A **regional flap** uses skin that is not right beside the area that requires a skin graft. The flap is stitched in place but remains attached by a narrow neck of tissue called a pedicle to its original source until the flap has healed into its new site, when the pedicle is removed.

SKIN GRAFTS

There are two main types of skin graft: a full thickness skin graft that includes the epidermis and the dermis below it, and a split thickness skin graft in which only the epidermis and upper dermis is used as a graft.

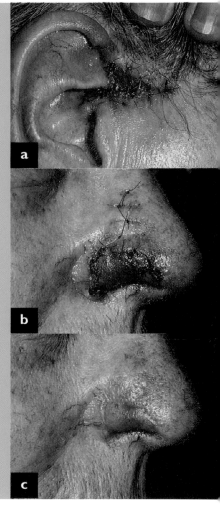

A full thickness skin graft

A month after surgery to remove a squamous cell carcinoma (see page 131), skin is taken from another site to replace the skin lost from the patient's nose.

a The donor site for the skin graft is just below the hairline, in front of an ear. Scarring in this area will not be noticeable.

b The donor skin is grafted over the scarred nostril. In this picture the skin graft has been in place for one week and the stitches are about to be taken out.

c Four weeks after surgery, the new graft has healed very well. The pink colouring should fade with time.

Full thickness skin graft

A full thickness skin graft is the best choice when cosmetic appearance (as on the face, for example) or the ability to stand up to wear and tear (as with the palm of the hand) are important factors. There is a limit to how much skin can be taken from the donor site, however, because skin at the donor site will not grow back: instead, the cut edges are stitched together to close the wound.

The surgeon tries to match skin from the donor site as closely as possible to the skin at the recipient site; sites chosen are generally free of terminal hairs, and have skin to spare (as in the crease of the elbow, for example).

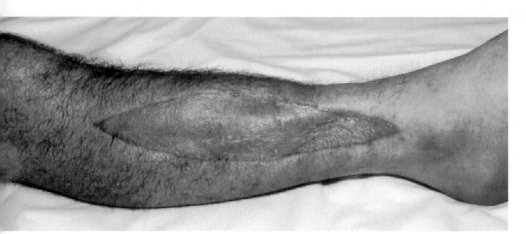

A split thickness skin graft
A skin graft such as the one shown in place here is performed when a wound is too large to be stitched shut or when severe scarring would occur if the wound was left to heal naturally.

Split thickness skin graft

With a split thickness graft, enough of the epidermal appendages (hair follicles and sweat and sebaceous glands) remain at the donor site for the skin to grow back and close the defect made by the graft. Therefore larger areas of skin can be taken from a donor site than would be possible with a full thickness graft – an entire thigh can be stripped if need be – and so larger areas of damaged skin can be covered than would be possible using a full thickness skin graft. The skin graft itself is a form of biological dressing; with time, the grafted skin is shed and the patient's own skin regenerates.

The disadvantage is that the donor site can be left very raw and sore for several weeks, until it eventually heals over. (Patients who have undergone split thickness skin grafts often suffer more pain from donor sites than do patients with full thickness skin grafts.) Also, the final result at the recipient site is frequently less satisfactory than after a full thickness graft: the new skin is likely to be less supple, hairless and not look so good.

Skin is shaved off the donor site using a power dermatome – a surgical instrument that cuts off very thin slices of skin – or a scalpel blade. The donor site most often used is the front of the thighs.

POSSIBLE COMPLICATIONS

- **Graft death** This can occur due to an infection, a small bleed below the skin graft, or a poor blood supply to the graft. A poor blood supply may be precipitated by a patient smoking, therefore patients are encouraged to give up smoking a week prior to surgery and for at least two weeks afterwards, whilst the graft is taking.
- **Graft may contract** Other complications related to skin grafts include the fact that sometimes the wound area contracts and shrinks in size, pulling on neighbouring

tissues and giving the skin a puckered appearance.
- **Sore donor site** For some patients the main problem is not so much the recipient site but the donor site, which can be sore and uncomfortable for some time after the graft has been removed. It is for this reason that local flaps have an obvious advantage.

SKIN TRANSPLANTS

When a patient has a wound that needs to be covered with skin at once, but not enough healthy skin for this job, the patient may receive skin from another donor (living or dead) as a temporary biological dressing. This solution has to be short-term because the patient's body will ultimately reject the 'foreign' skin, and the use of immunosuppressive drugs to prevent rejection is not a suitable treatment for someone who has a major skin defect and is therefore wide open to infection. Cadaver skin (generally from the thighs and back) can be stored in a skin bank, if this facility is available. Britain's first skin bank, the Stephen Kirby Skin Bank at Queen Mary's Hospital in Roehampton, London, opened in 1995.

AT THE LEADING EDGE

Growing new skin for grafting

One solution to the problem of finding a supply of suitable skin for permanent grafting is to grow new skin. To avoid rejection by the patient's body, the new skin needs to be 'grown' from a sample taken from the patient's own body. Scientists can now do this for the epidermis at least. They can take a strip of epidermis the size of a postage stamp and stimulate the cells to multiply, producing a sheet of epidermal skin that can be grafted over the patient's wound. But at present the process is a slow and expensive one, and so this treatment is not yet as widely available as doctors would like.

Treatments for burns

When dealing with a burn, the first priority is to prevent infection from taking hold in the damaged area. Then healing must be promoted by whatever means is most appropriate. In serious burns, overcoming shock is often an immediate and pressing concern.

The causes of burns are: fire, water (scalding), chemicals, electricity and UVR. A burn's seriousness depends on how much of the surface area of the skin is affected as well as how deeply a burn has penetrated the skin.

SHOCK

Swelling and blistering result from leakage of plasma from blood vessels damaged by a burn. In burns affecting 15 per cent or more of skin surface in adults (10 per cent in children) loss of plasma impairs the circulation, leading to shock and requiring an immediate blood or saline transfusion to restore the blood volume.

Pain-killing drugs are also important, since pain contributes to shock. Loss of nerve-endings in the deeper layers of the skin can result in a third-degree burn being less painful than a first or second-degree burn.

INFECTION

An ever-present danger with burns of any sort is infection. To lower the risk of infection, antibiotics are often prescribed.

Different depths of burn

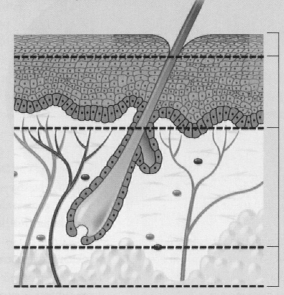

First-degree burn
Affects superficial cells of the epidermis

Superficial second-degree burn
Damages epidermis and upper dermis

Deep second-degree burn
Affects the epidermis and deep dermis

Third-degree burn
The epidermis and dermis are destroyed and tissues below are also affected

SKIN HEALING AND REPAIR

Treatment varies according to the depth and extent of the burn.
- **First-degree burns** may require no special treatment apart from initial cooling of the burn by prolonged immersion in cool, clean water.
- **Second-degree burns** may fully heal, provided that traces of sebaceous and sweat glands and hair follicles remain within the dermis and there

is no extra damage from infection. A dressing will keep the area moist and prevent infection. Often a topical agent is applied as well.
- **Third-degree burns** are often severe enough to require a skin graft. The hair follicles and sweat glands have been destroyed and so the skin cannot grow back, unless it is able to grow inwards from the edges of the wound.

Mesh skin graft

a A piece of skin taken from an unburnt donor site on the patient is prepared for a skin graft by being passed through a mesh machine. This enlarges it considerably by turning it into a hexagonal lattice.

b The mesh skin graft is laid over the burn injury and held in place with a dressing. This technique can be used when burns are so extensive there is not enough healthy skin remaining for a traditional skin graft.

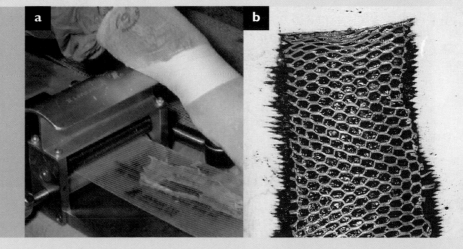

Laser treatments for skin conditions

Lasers allow the destruction of the target tissue only, with surrounding tissues remaining intact and bleeding kept to a minimum. In recent years these advantages has been put to use to treat various lesions and vascular conditions, and the effects of sun damage and ageing.

Depending on the power, wavelength, exposure time and tissue being targeted, lasers can have several different effects on the body, hence their use in many different clinical specialties. In dermatology they are most used for their heat-producing effects.

The type of laser and its optimal wavelength dictate its use: alexandrite and ruby lasers, for example, target melanin so are used to treat pigment problems; carbon dioxide lasers vaporise tissue so are used in skin resurfacing or cutting; bromide and argon lasers target haemoglobin so are used to treat problems in blood vessels or to heat seal vessels.

LASERS FOR VASCULAR SKIN CONDITIONS

Conditions that are vascular are those related to or supplied with blood vessels. They include facial thread veins, and birthmarks such as port wine stains and strawberry naevi. Lasers to treat vascular conditions

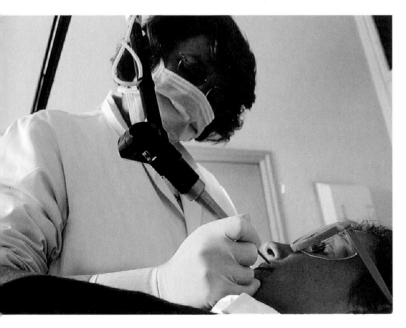

Laser treatment in action
The laser works by focusing extreme light and heat energy on a very small area, vaporising that area in the process. The energy is emitted from the needle-like device at centre and is visible as a red dot on the face of the patient.

Is laser therapy the best way of treating thread veins in the legs?

For thread veins – broken blood vessels – in the lower legs the traditional treatment is sclerotherapy. The veins are injected with sclerosant chemicals that cause the veins to shrivel and close down, thus improving their appearance. In recent years laser treatments have been introduced, but experience has revealed that laser therapy for thread veins in the legs is not as effective as sclerotherapy.

ASK THE EXPERT

target the red of haemoglobin in blood cells, leading to heat generation and the destruction of blood vessels. The first lasers were painful for patients and resulted in bruising. These older lasers have largely been superseded by lasers with associated cooling devices to allow the top layer of the skin to remain undamaged by the heat generated by the laser. Cooling the skin ahead of time and during the procedure also reduces pain for the patient. In addition, these newer lasers produce less bruising and can penetrate deeper into the skin, allowing the treatment of deeper blood vessels or other vascular lesions.

Laser therapy for facial thread veins

Thread veins are broken blood vessels that are visible because they are so close to the skin's surface. The most common cause of facial thread veins is overexposure to ultraviolet radiation (UVR). Facial thread veins used to be treated with electrocautery, but there was always a risk that a patient would be left with a small depressed scar. Today, laser therapy is the preferred treatment. Lasers used to treat vascular skin conditions are very effective tools for removing facial blood vessels, leaving minimal bruising. However, there is a small risk that the facial thread veins will return in a few years time. It may be that this happens when UVR is the underlying cause, and recurrence occurs with repeated exposure to UVR.

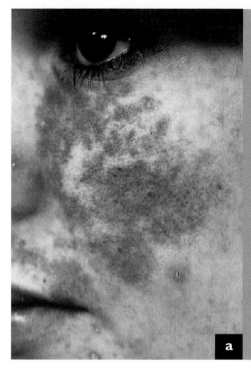

Lightening a birthmark

a An increase in the size of blood vessels in the skin results in a port wine stain, an area of permanent flushing. In children, these stains are flat and pink but they become more purple with age. They may also become more 'lumpy', which can make applying camouflage makeup difficult (the British Red Cross offers advice on skin camouflage, see page 160). Treatment using an argon laser can be very successful.

b Up to 10 treatment sessions about 8 weeks apart produce significant skin lightening in up to 90 per cent of affected individuals.

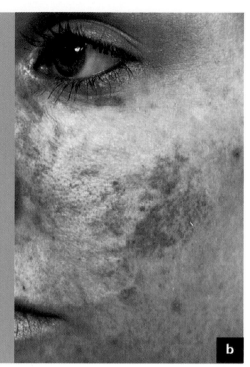

ABLATIVE LASERS

Ablative lasers are destructive: they vaporise or remove skin, and can also cut tissue quickly and precisely. They can treat blood vessel problems and excess pigmentation, remove warts and skin tags, or resurface the skin following acne, sun damage or signs of ageing. With each pass of the laser over the skin, the skin is removed. Bleeding is kept to a minimum, which limits blood loss and allowing the operator a clearer view of the operation site.

The main advantage of laser ablation for skin resurfacing is its success rate: by removing the top layer of skin, leaving unblemished skin beneath, the appearance of the skin is often dramatically improved. There are many disadvantages, however, including:

• Healing can take up to six months.
• The skin can be left with prolonged redness and occasionally some discoloration. Although temporary, this inflammation can be uncomfortable or even painful for patients.
• Patients may be unable to go to work for several weeks after the procedure, while the skin is healing.
• Because the skin is raw after surgery it is prone to infection; often patients are given antibiotics or antiviral treatment to lower the risk of acquiring an infection.
• Patients with darker skins are often left with permanently discoloured skin.

NON-ABLATIVE LASERS

A non-ablative laser, by definition, does not vaporise the skin. These lasers are used at a lower wavelength than ablative models, and so don't produce heat. They can treat facial lines caused by ageing and sun damage, and also soft scarring. They act by stimulating collagen production, thereby 'plumping' the skin up so that slight irregularities are softened and the skin's appearance is improved.

Non-ablative lasers have several advantages over conventional resurfacing lasers:

• They may be used on patients of all skin types.
• Because there is no skin ablation, there is no recovery time; sometimes patients have this treatment and go straight back to work.

The disadvantages are that improvements in appearance may take place more slowly and be more subtle.

LASERS FOR OTHER SKIN CONDITIONS

Lasers are also now available to treat pigmented growths such as seborrhoeic warts (basal cell papillomas, see page 136). They have also been modified to remove tattoos, as well as pigment changes. Laser tattoo removal has mixed results: some pigments respond better than others, so a tattoo that is primarily black or blue is fairly easy to remove completely, while reds and yellows are more difficult. Laser tattoo removal should not leave any scar.

Mohs micrographic surgery

In the 1950s, Dr Frederick Mohs developed a technique for excising basal cell carcinomas and similar tumours. Mohs micrographic surgery (MMS) has been refined and improved ever since and is now a sophisticated, widely used technique.

Basal cell carcinoma (BCC) is the most common form of cancer in both the United States of America and Australia, and is showing an increase in incidence in the UK. It occurs almost exclusively in white-skinned people and the most significant causative factor is continued exposure over time to sunlight. For this reason it occurs mainly in the areas of the body that are exposed – the head, neck and face. BCCs tend to be relatively slow growing and not to spread to other parts of the body. The aim of treatment is to preserve as much healthy surrounding skin and tissue as possible. It involves the alternate removal and microscopic examination of any tissue harbouring cancer cells. It results in the total eradication of the cancer.

This type of surgery is generally performed by dermatologists and plastic surgeons in the UK, and a patient may be referred to either of these specialists. However, if the BCC is moderate to large in size, it may be that a plastic surgeon is best qualified to repair or reconstruct the skin after surgery.

For many plastic surgeons and dermatologists, MMS is the gold standard of treatment for BCCs, particularly those around the eyes and nose. Other treatments – such as cryosurgery, curettage and cautery, radiotherapy and topical therapy with drugs – may also be used, but they have the disadvantage of not detecting that all cancer cells have been removed. There is, therefore, a significant risk of recurrence. Other cancers that might be treated by MMS include squamous cell carcinomas and some small malignant melanomas.

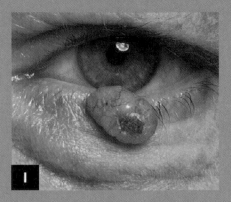

1

The procedure – step by step

1 MMS is a good treatment option for a cancer in an area where it is important to preserve healthy tissue for functional and aesthetic reasons, such as around the eyes. The procedure involves alternate surgery and microscopic examination of removed tissue to detect the 'roots' of the visible cancer. The patient is given a local anaesthetic and may also be sedated.

2 The visible tumour is removed and examined under a microscope. The surgeon builds up a 'site map' of the tumour, detecting areas where there are still cancer roots in the skin. Using the 'map', the surgeon returns to an area where cancerous cells remain, and removes a thin layer of tissue. This is examined under the microscope. If any area of removed tissue still shows signs of cancer, the surgeon returns to that area and removes another thin slice of tissue for microscopic examination. This continues until no cancerous cells can be detected.

3 Removal of only cancerous tissue preserves as much normal tissue as possible, while still enabling the surgeon to be sure that the horizontal and vertical margins of the incisions are clear of cancer. The surgeon then chooses the best healing option for the patient.

4 The wound heals to be barely noticeable.

Advantages of MMS

- The doctor can be sure that all of the cancer cells have been taken away, because the whole cancer is excised and examined in its entirety rather than in small sections. This minimises the chances of false negative results.
- The size of the remaining hole and hence the scar will be smaller because the doctor does not have to estimate the extent of the malignant growth.
- The surgery can generally be performed under a local anaesthetic in an outpatient clinic,

which means that even elderly and frail patients who might not be well enough for a general anaesthetic, can benefit from the surgery.
- The surgery is successful, with an overall five-year cure rate of 99 per cent.
- Mohs is not suitable for everyone. The most likely candidates have a recurrence of a BCC more than 2cm (¾in) in diameter on the eyes, ears, lips or nose, or on the nose to mouth lines (nasolabial folds). A BCC invading surrounding nerves may also be treated with MMS.

How MMS works

Once the visible tumour has been removed (stage one), it is quartered, then sliced horizontally: each slice is analysed under the microscope. From this, the surgeon can build up a 'map' of the contours of the tumour (stage two). Tissue is removed from targeted cancerous areas, sliced and examined and more cancerous cells are removed (stage three). The procedure continues until all cancerous cells have been removed (stage four).

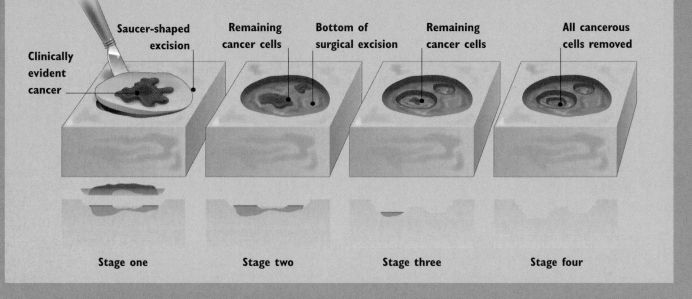

Clinically evident cancer | Saucer-shaped excision | Remaining cancer cells | Bottom of surgical excision | Remaining cancer cells | All cancerous cells removed

Stage one　　**Stage two**　　**Stage three**　　**Stage four**

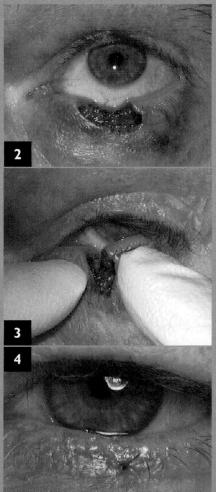

HEALING AFTER MMS

Healing is dependent upon the size of the original tumour. Occasionally the wound may be left to heal on its own. When very small growths (less than 1cm/½in) are excised, the edges of the wound will probably be stitched together. If stitches are used, they will be removed after 5–10 days, depending on the site. There will initially be a red scar, but this will gradually fade. It is important to protect the scar from further sun damage and a sunblock should be used over it at all times to prevent it from over-growing (a so-called hypertrophic scar).

When larger growths are removed, a skin graft may be taken from another part of the body – usually an area that is not seen, such as the buttock or thigh – to fill the gap. Dressings will be applied and checked regularly until the patient's own skin has has had time to grow over and fill the gap.

Occasionally, it may not be possible to fill the defect with a skin graft. In this case a plastic surgeon will create a skin flap – a small area of skin that is moved, along with its blood supply, from an area near to the wound site. Very good cosmetic results can be achieved with this technique, although this may not always be immediately apparent. It is important that patients ask their surgeon to show them photographs of previous surgeries for reassurance.

In the right hands, MMS is a highly effective method for treating basal cell and other carcinomas, and patients heal well. However, it should only be performed by doctors who have been specially trained and are experienced in the procedure.

Treating skin cancer

Although the majority of skin cancers are not fatal, they do cause disfiguring growths which can increase in size and destroy local structures in the skin. Early detection and management of such growths is of paramount importance.

Skin cancers can arise from any component of the skin, including the blood vessels, sweat glands, nerve fibres, fatty tissue and muscle wall. However, all these skin cancers are relatively rare. For example, mycoides fungoides, which has an effect on the skin via the immune system, affects less than one in 10,000 people. By far the commonest forms of skin cancer – basal cell carcinomas, squamous cell carcinomas and malignant melanomas – arise from the epidermis of the skin.

SUN AND SKIN CANCER

There is increasing public awareness that one of the main causes of skin cancer is excess exposure to ultraviolet radiation (UVR) from the sun, hence the tendency of cancerous growths to develop on parts of the body most often exposed to sunlight, such as the face, hands and shoulders. People with very fair skins and those prone to sunburn are most at risk. Although it is true that incidences of skin cancer are higher in countries with lots of sunlight such as Australia and South Africa, it is important to remember that it is UV exposure that is the risk factor, and UV light can penetrate through clouds.

BASAL CELL CARCINOMA (BCC)

The commonest form of skin cancer is a basal cell carcinoma. It is sometimes referred to as a rodent ulcer because the growth does not spread elsewhere in the body but very slowly nibbles away at local tissue in a rodent-like manner. The outlook for a patient with a BCC is good as it does not spread to other areas of the body. If left untreated, however, a BCC can disfigure, and so early recognition and treatment are important. There are about 40,000 cases of BCCs each year in the UK alone.

There is no doubt that a major cause of BCCs is long-term exposure to sunlight. They are more frequently seen in patients over the age of 50, but now younger and younger people are developing such cancers, reflecting changes in attitudes and habits regarding sun exposure.

A rodent ulcer may first come to the patient's notice as a skin lesion or sore that fails to heal within a month or so, or that bleeds spontaneously. It can be flesh coloured, pink, red or brown like a mole. It can begin as a red patch, or as a flat scarred area on the skin that may appear pale or white compared to the surrounding skin.

Treatment of a basal cell carcinoma

Management of these tumours depends to some extent upon the type of tumour present, where it is located, its size, and the general health of the patient.

- **Curettage and cautery** This is the process of surgically removing the tumour by scraping away the surrounding tissue and then cauterising the base as a way both of stopping bleeding and of destroying any tumour cells that may remain in the skin. This has a high cure rate and produces a very satisfactory cosmetic result.
- **Cryotherapy using liquid nitrogen** Freezing the BCC and thereby inducing a degree of cell damage and necrosis produces a good result for many patients, particularly

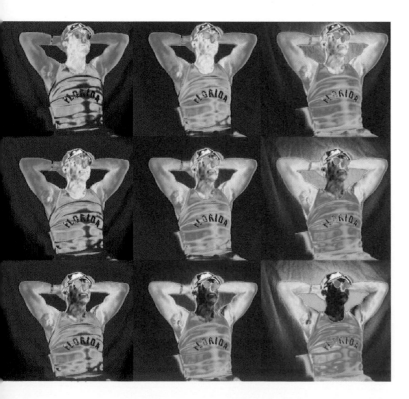

The effect of the sun on skin temperature
A thermogram uses photographic film sensitive to UVR to measure the heat given off various parts of the body. The man's face starts off cool (yellow to green, 30–32°C, top left) but soon becomes much hotter (red, 35°C, bottom right).

Radiotherapy for a basal cell carcinoma

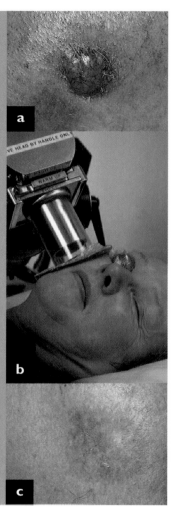

a This red ulcer-like growth is a basal cell carcinoma on the face. It started as a small, flat nodule, then slowly broke down in the centre to form a shallow ulcer.

b Here it is being treated by radiotherapy. The patient has lead blocks (covered with cling film) on her eye and cheek to protect healthy cells from the radiation. The machine focuses X-rays on the BCC, which slow or stop altogether the growth of abnormal cells,

c Three months after radiotherapy treatment, the BCC has gone and only a pink patch remains.

those with growths on the back. A disadvantage is that the freezing often produces a wound that can take from a few weeks to a few months to heal fully.

- **Ablative laser therapy** For patients with a number of BCCs on the trunk and back, a carbon dioxide laser can be an effective, rapid treatment. It removes tissue and keeps bleeding to a minimum. Unfortunately there is as yet little data on this therapy's long-term effectiveness.

- **Excision of the actual growth** The growth on the skin is cut out and then the defect is closed up with sutures. Alternatively, a flap made of local skin may be used (see page 121) or a skin graft if the defect is very large.

- **Radiotherapy** Many dermatology centres now have combined clinics where a dermatologist, radiotherapist and surgeon decide together on the best treatment for each patient. For some patients the demands of frequent attendance at the centre for radiotherapy sessions can be a problem. There is also the disadvantage that

scarring can initially look fairly acceptable, but years later there may be some significant appearance of scar tissue and broken blood vessels at the site of treatment.

- **Topical therapy** The use of a cream such as 5 Flurouracil can produce a good cure for BCCs, especially those on the lower legs, where surgery or radiotherapy would not be advisable because these areas can heal poorly.

- **Photodynamic therapy** Many centres have reported some good results with this treatment. The combined use of a cream and light source produce cell destruction at the tumour site (see page 111). The cosmetic results can be excellent. Evidence to date suggests that the risk of recurrence is similar to that of other treatments, although long-term data has yet to be published.

- **Mohs micrographic surgery** has been around for many years (see page 128).

What are the chances of a second BCC?

It has been estimated that 40 per cent of patients will develop a new BCC within 5 years of the first. With this in mind, anyone who has developed a BCC should do what they can to reduce the chances of this happening by limiting their sun exposure, wearing adequate sun protection when they do go out in the sun and checking their skin on a regular basis for any suspicious lesions.

SQUAMOUS CELL CARCINOMA (SCC)

The second most common type of skin cancer in the UK is a squamous cell carcinoma. Often an SCC takes the form of a lump, which may ulcerate, become crusty and bleed, and be quite painful to touch. There is a small risk of such a tumour spreading to another part of the body. It is estimated that about 10,000 SCCs are diagnosed every year in the UK and the number is increasing.

The development of a squamous cell carcinoma is usually related to chronic UV exposure, much like BCCs, and therefore SCCs too are especially common on the sun-damaged skin of fair-skinned people. Alternatively, an SCC may develop as a result of previous exposure to radiation, in a patient who has a chronic wound in the skin, or in a patient who has impaired immune function.

Treatment of a squamous cell carcinoma

The main aims of treatment are the destruction of the primary growth and the prevention of the tumour spreading elsewhere. The earlier the diagnosis and treatment, the better.

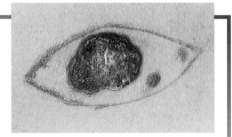

REMOVAL OF A MALIGNANT MELANOMA

I only mentioned to my GP in passing the appearance of a small dark mole on my tummy. He booked me into the local dermatology clinic 'just in case'.

Here, after examining the mole, the dermatologist said she wanted to remove the mole that very afternoon. The operation began with a local anaesthetic by injection, then the doctor made two curved incisions into the skin on either side of the mole. The mole was taken out and the cut secured with a few stitches. The whole procedure was quite painless.

The mole was sent off for biopsy. A week later I received the bad news that it was a malignant melanoma. I returned to the clinic the next day, when more of the area around the mole was cut away – again under local anaesthetic. Since then there has been no sign of the cancer spreading – I have been very lucky.

- **Surgical excision** is the treatment of choice, depending on the patient's age and health, and the site of the tumour.
- **Curettage and cautery** can produce a very good result.
- **Radiotherapy** can be effective.
- **Mohs micrographic surgery** has been used for the management of squamous cell carcinomas.

Treatment is followed up with regular skin surveillance and advice to the patient on adequate sun protection.

MALIGNANT MELANOMA

The most worrying type of skin malignancy is a malignant melanoma. It is estimated that between four and five thousand melanomas are diagnosed every year in the UK.

A malignant melanoma can occur spontaneously, or develop from a pre-existing mole. In terms of the risk of developing a malignant melanoma, it is not so much chronic ultraviolet exposure as periods of sunburn, particularly in childhood, that appear to be important.

Occasionally a malignant melanoma develops from a mole that was present at birth (the vast majority of moles appear during childhood and adolescence).

Treatment of a malignant melanoma

As with other skin cancers, the aim is early detection and early management. Any change in a mole's condition (see page 107) should be reported to the GP immediately.

- **Surgery** The principle treatment for malignant melanoma remains surgical intervention. The mole is removed together with a safety margin of skin around the mole to ensure, as far as possible, that all the cancerous cells have been removed.
- **Regular monitoring** After the mole has been removed, a patient is given a full skin check at regular intervals to be sure that the growth has not reappeared in the scar itself or anywhere else. These checks take place for at least five years after the operation. In addition, patients are taught how to examine their own skin thoroughly so they too can look out for suspicious growths.

The trend in recent years is that patients and doctors between them are picking up more malignant melanomas much earlier than previously, which leads to a better outcome for more patients. If a malignant melanoma recurs, further surgery, chemotherapy, radiotherapy and vaccination therapy (the injection of antigens to stimulate the immune system to fight the cancer cells) are all possibilities.

Squamous carcinoma cells
An immunofluorescent light micrograph shows squamous carcinoma cells cultured from a tumour.

A to Z

OF DISEASES AND DISORDERS

This section gives information on the main illnesses and medical conditions that can affect the skin, hair and nails.

This index is arranged alphabetically and each entry is structured in a similar way:

What are the causes?

What are the symptoms?

How is it diagnosed?

What are the treatment options?

What is the outlook?

ACNE

A condition in which excess sebum and a growth change in cells in the hair follicle leads to blockage of skin pores. These can become inflamed and infected appearing as spots on the skin.

What are the causes?

This very common condition is a disorder of the hair follicles and associated sebaceous glands, which produce sebum. Excess production is triggered by hormonal changes at puberty, and there may be a family history of acne.

What are the symptoms?

A variety of skin lesions are seen – ranging from non-inflamed blackheads and whiteheads, to inflamed papules and pustules, through to large nodular lesions and cysts. The larger lesions may leave scarring once healed.

Acne commonly affects the face, back, shoulders and chest and ranges in severity from mild to severe. It can be a distressing condition for the self-conscious teenager, and also in adults who feel they should have grown out of it.

What are the treatment options?

In mild acne, creams or lotions applied directly to the affected areas (known as 'topical' treatments) may be sufficient. These preparations can be antibiotics or agent that unblock skin pores, or a combination of the two.

DEFINITIONS

BIOPSY Removal of a piece of skin under local anaesthetic for diagnostic purposes.

ERYTHEMA Used in dermatology to mean redness of the skin.

EXCORIATIONS Breaks in the skin surface caused by scratching.

LESION General term used to indicate any abnormality of the skin.

MACULE A flat area of altered skin.

NODULE A large papule.

PAPULE Small raised bump on the skin surface.

PATCH Flat area of affected skin, larger than a macule.

PLAQUE A patch which is raised above the surface level of the skin.

PUSTULE A papule containing pus.

SEBUM Oily substance produced by sebaceous glands within the skin.

In more serious cases, tablet treatments are used. Females can use a particular form of the oral contraceptive pill, which helps due to its hormonal action. In both males and females antibiotics are helpful when used regularly for at least six months. These should be used in combination with a topical vitamin A drug to unblock the pores.

In severe acne, isotretinoin is a treatment option. This is a course of tablets for at least four months, available through hospital dermatologists. Blood tests are required before and during treatment, and since fetal abnormalities can result from taking this drug, effective contraception must be in place before it starts. The drug has been implicated in depression and suicide attempts, and this risk must be made known to the patient and parents. Phototherapy (p. 112) can help, and larger cysts may be settled with steroid injections.

No matter what the severity, regular gentle cleansing of the face is recommended. It is unlikely that any change in diet will improve the condition.

The majority of people will be clear of acne by their mid 20s, but it can persist in some to the 30s, 40s and beyond.

ACTINIC (SOLAR) KERATOSES

These can be pre-malignant lesions, not in themselves cancerous, but they may become so if left untreated.

What are the causes?

As the name suggests this condition arises due to excess sun exposure with inadequate protection.

What are the symptoms?

These lesions may be present singly or in large numbers and are most common in the fair skinned. Men are affected more frequently than women. They appear as warty papules or patches, with a rough, scaly surface. They may be pink, grey or brown and are usually asymptomatic. The face, scalp, ears and back of hands are most commonly affected.

How is it diagnosed?

They are generally diagnosed on appearance, but a biopsy can be performed if necessary.

What are the treatment options?

Anyone with solar keratoses should cover up in the sun and use a sunscreen on any exposed areas of skin.

Individual lesions can be treated with cryotherapy (p. 119), but if large areas are affected, particularly on the face, this may not be practical. Regular application of a topical chemotherapy cream for four weeks may settle them over 2–3 months. Particularly stubborn lesions or those with doubtful diagnosis can be removed under local anaesthetic.

What is the outlook?
There is a small risk that keratoses can become cancerous, so any areas which are changing or not responding to treatment should be reported to your doctor. Also, people affected by solar keratoses are at an increased risk of other sun-related skin cancers, and should get new or suspicious areas checked by their doctor sooner rather than later.

ALBINISM
A condition characterised by hereditary lack of pigment.

What are the causes?
Albinism is a genetically transmitted condition occurring in roughly 1 in 20,000 people in Britain. A defect in pigment production leads to white/pink skin, blonde or white hair, and lack of colour in the eyes. Those affected tolerate sun poorly as they burn easily, and often have poor eyesight.

How is it diagnosed?
Diagnosis can be made in the uterus with fetal skin biopsy, and this may be indicated in tropical countries. After birth the diagnosis is apparent without investigation.

What are the treatment options?
The main treatment is sun avoidance through regular use of at least a SPF 50 sunblock and sun-protective clothing.

What is the outlook?
A small amount of pigment may appear with age.
In temperate climates, the prognosis is good: people with albinism can live relatively normally. In the tropics, early development of skin cancers makes the outlook less good.

ALOPECIA AREATA
Loss of hair in discrete coin-shaped areas.

What are the causes?
This is thought to be due to an exaggerated immune response targeted against the hair root. There may be a background of affected family members, and in some cases it seems to follow emotional or physical trauma.

What are the symptoms?
Rounded patches of hair loss are seen, with a distinct edge and normal skin on the exposed scalp. It usually starts to appear in the teens and 20s. Hair can be plucked for analysis or a biopsy taken if there is any doubt of the diagnosis.

What are the treatment options?
If the patch is fairly small and causing no concern, no treatment is needed. For larger areas, steroids can be used either as a lotion or injected into the affected skin. Phototherapy may be helpful in severe cases. In 70–80 per cent of cases, hair regrowth – usually white – occurs without treatment, although recurrent episodes are not unusual. A small percentage may progress to total hair loss.

BASAL CELL CARCINOMA (BCC)
The most common form of skin cancer.

What are the causes?
BCC affects males more often than females, especially on the face. Like many skin cancers, it is most commonly due to sun exposure over many years. It is thought that excess sun up to the age of 20 is the most important factor, although BCCs generally do not develop until middle age or later.

What are the symptoms?
There are different types of BCC. The most common tends to start as a slow-growing nodule with a pearly edge containing visible blood vessels. As it grows – which is a slow process – it tends to ulcerate in the centre – hence the alternative name 'rodent ulcer'. ('Rodent' because if left it eats away slowly at the surrounding skin and tissues.) The next most common type is a red scaly plaque which slowly increases in size. It lies more superficially in the skin, hence the name superficial BCC. In a third type, morphoeic BCC, the cancer cells induce a reaction in the skin with the production of almost a scar. The skin feels firm and may have blood vessels on the surface.

The appearance suggests the diagnosis, which is confirmed by biopsy.

What are the treatment options?
Removal under local anaesthetic is the likely treatment. Freezing with liquid nitrogen is sometimes successful for superficial tumours, and photodynamic therapy is becoming common (p. 111).

What is the outlook?
The outlook for BCC is very good as it does not spread to other areas of the body. Having had one nodule increases the risk of developing more, so regular check-ups and avoidance of excess sun are essential.

BASAL CELL PAPILLOMA
An extremely common benign skin condition, also known as a seborrhoeic wart.

Typically these are greasy, brown lesions with a warty surface which look as if they have been stuck on to the skin, but the colour can vary from pink to black. They are seen mainly after 40 years of age, and any site can be affected. Some people may have one or two but some have dozens, in varying sizes. The cause is unknown: genetics, viral infection or sun exposure may play a part. No treatment is necessary as these are benign, not infectious and have no effect on health. However they may be unsightly or catch on clothing, in which case they can be frozen with liquid nitrogen (p. 119). Particularly large warts can be removed under local anaesthetic if necessary.

BIRTHMARKS
Common skin markings which vary in severity from minor to disfiguring – not all are present from birth.

CAPILLARY HAEMANGIOMA
Also known as strawberry naevus, these appear in the first four weeks of life as a tiny red spot, and grow over a few weeks to produce a deep red swelling, composed of blood vessels, with a soft, spongy feel. One in five infants have more than one. These resolve with age – 50 per cent are gone within five years and 75 per cent by seven years. If affecting vision or feeding, or if bleeding excessively, systemic steroids, surgery or laser treatment may be needed.

EPIDERMAL NAEVUS
Present from birth or developing later in adulthood, this has a warty or velvety appearance. They can be removed by cryotherapy (p. 119) or laser therapy (p. 126–7).

CONGENITAL MELANOCYTIC NAEVUS (MOLE)
Ten per cent of the population are born with one or more moles. These start as flat circular or oval areas of pigmentation, but often change in appearance at puberty.

They may become raised or slightly warty. Normal moles have an even colour and even border. Large moles or those sited in awkward places can be removed. See Moles (p. 147).

MONGOLIAN SPOT
A bluish-black birthmark on the lower back, most common in Asian/African races, which clears in later childhood.

NAEVUS FLAMMEUS
Also known as port wine stains, these darker red/purplish patches are seen on the face or upper body. They tend to affect one side of the body and do not cross the midline. Those around the eye may extend internally and can cause epilepsy. They do not resolve without treatment, but can respond to laser treatment or be covered with cosmetics.

SALMON PATCH
Also known as stork marks these pinkish-red patches on the forehead and/or back of the neck are very common. Salmon patches on the forehead usually resolve over a few years; those on the neck tend to remain into adulthood.

SEBACEOUS NAEVUS
A hairless red/orange plaque on the scalp, which may grow and become warty at puberty. Skin cancer can develop in these birthmarks, so they should be monitored or removed.

BLISTERS
Blisters are caused by an accumulation of fluid within the top layers of the skin.

Small blisters are known as 'vesicles', larger ones as 'bullae'. There are a number of causes of blistering disorders including infection (chickenpox and shingles, for example), dermatitis, trauma, bites, sunburn, medicines and autoimmune diseases such as pemphigoid/pemphigus (p. 150). Treatment depends on the underlying cause.

BOILS
A boil is tender, red skin nodule, caused by infection of a hair follicle with Staphylococcus bacteria.

After about a week pus is visible under the skin; this can be painful and swollen until the boil bursts and the pus drains away. Keeping the area clean and applying warm compresses several times a day to bring the boil to a head are usually all that is required. However, large painful boils can be lanced by a doctor. Occasionally antibiotics can limit the spread of infection. A furuncle is another term for boil; a collection of boils is a carbuncle.

BOWEN'S DISEASE
A pre-cancerous condition which progresses slowly.

What are the causes?
Bowen's disease can be caused by excess sun exposure, and has been linked to arsenic ingestion. Cancerous cells may be seen under microscopic examination. They are confined to the surface of the skin, and are generally easily treated.

What are the symptoms?
Typically, Bowen's disease is found on the shins of middle aged to elderly women, although men may be affected, and it may also be seen elsewhere on the body. It appears as a dark pink scaly patch with a distinct edge, but generally does not cause any other symptoms. It may take years to become a few centimetres in diameter.

What are the treatment options?
If the patch is quite small, it can be removed under local anaesthetic. However, cryotherapy (p. 119) is often sufficient. Photodynamic therapy (p. 111) is increasingly being used. Your doctor may also prescribe treatment in a cream form (5-fluorouracil). Although very slow growing if left untreated, Bowen's disease does have the potential to develop into squamous cell carcinoma (p. 154) so treatment is required once it has been detected.

CAMPBELL DE MORGAN SPOTS
These common skin lesions are due to an overgrowth of small blood vessels in the skin.

These lesions appear as bright red papules particularly on the trunk in the middle aged and elderly. No treatment is necessary as the condition is benign.

CELLULITIS
An acute bacterial infection of the skin.

Although it can happen to anyone, diabetics or those with poor circulation are more likely to develop cellulitis, in which the skin becomes red, hot, swollen and tender, often with painful enlargement of nearby lymph nodes. There may be an obvious entry for the infection such as a bite or cut. Antibiotics are used to clear the infection, either orally or intravenously, depending on the severity. Some individuals may have recurrent episodes.

Necrotising fasciitis is a particularly aggressive type of cellulitis in which the affected area becomes dusky, blistered and numb. If left untreated the affected skin and underlying tissue eventually dies off.

CHICKENPOX
A very common viral infection, particularly in children, caused by infection with the varicella zoster virus, a type of herpes virus.

What are the symptoms?
The rash consists of small blisters which burst and crust over, and may heal to leave small white scars. It is itchy and the whole body may be affected. It may be preceded by cold symptoms. Diagnosis is made on appearance.

What are the treatment options?
Generally no treatment is needed. Bathing and the use of calamine lotion can help to relieve the itch. Chickenpox is contagious until the spots dry (and for several days before they appear). The incubation period is about 14 days. Chickenpox is rarely caught more than once, although shingles may develop years after chickenpox infection. Pregnant women who have not previously had chickenpox should contact their GP if exposed, as there is a risk to the unborn baby and vaccination may be required.

CHILBLAINS (PERNIOSIS)
Purple-pink swellings particularly on the fingers, toes and ears that result from exposure to cold weather.

Chilblains are a common condition, due to exaggerated 'shut down' of blood vessels in response to cold. They are more common in females and the elderly – possibly because they do not wrap up well enough in cold weather – and can be painful and itchy. Symptoms tend to be worse when warming up after exposure to the cold. Avoidance of cold is the main treatment. Weak steroid creams, or medicines which open up the blood vessels, may help. Chilblains settle in time, but recurrences are common.

CHONDRODERMATITIS NODULARIS HELICIS CHRONICUS (CDNHC)
Painful nodules on the outer ear due to inflammation of the cartilage.

The trigger for this painful condition, which may cause sleep disturbance if the nodules are rolled on during the night, is probably pressure on the ear during sleep. They are diagnosed on appearance. Treatment is usually in the form of removal under local anaesthetic, although cryotherapy (p. 119) may be used. The condition may recur, in which case a protective mould can be made to relieve pressure on the nodule, thereby avoiding further surgery.

CONTACT DERMATITIS
An allergic or irritant reaction to one or more environmental triggers.

What are the causes?
The condition is caused by external substances contacting the skin and causing eczema. The substances may be irritants (which would cause a similar reaction in anyone with ongoing exposure to the irritant) or allergens (which cause an allergic reaction only in susceptible individuals). In addition, irritant reactions tend to be gradual in onset, whereas allergic reactions are more immediate. Nickel is the most common cause of skin allergy, but glues, leathers, dyes, cosmetics, creams, chemicals and detergents may all cause irritant reactions.

Stainless steel's structure is such that the nickel it contains does not leach out on to the skin, so people with contact dermatitis can wear stainless steel jewellery or watch straps.

What are the symptoms?
The hands and face are commonly involved, but the site will depend on the area of the body which is in contact with the trigger. Nickel, found in a wide range of jewellery and other products, may cause a reaction on the ears or neck, or other areas where the skin is exposed: studs in clothing, for example, can affect the lower abdomen.

Some allergies are only activated when exposed to sunlight, a phenomenon known as photodermatitis.

How is it diagnosed?
Often individuals will recognise a trigger at work or in the home. However, patch testing is sometimes used to identify the cause of allergic dermatitis. This involves the application of small amounts of common allergens to the back for 48 hours (p. 109), then removing and looking for any reaction two days later.

What are the treatment options?
The main treatment is avoidance of identified irritants or allergens. Protective clothing may be necessary (for example, for mechanics with hand-contact dermatitis). Treatment is the same as for eczema. If known allergens or irritants can be avoided, the skin should settle.

CYST
A fluid-filled 'walled' lesion deep within the dermis.

It is still unclear why cysts appear: some babies are born with one or more, there may be a family history of the problem and they are more likely in smokers. Small cysts do not need treatment, but larger ones will be removed. Removal involves cutting out the whole cyst, including the wall, then stitching the wound. Cysts can however recur. If a cyst becomes infected, antibiotics may be necessary.

DERMATITIS ARTEFACTA
These are self-inflicted skin lesions.

The lesions are often bizarre in both shape and appearance and tend to be found on accessible areas. Often teenage girls/young women are affected, and there may be other evidence of psychological distress. Sufferers generally deny having any part in the condition and doctors base a diagnosis on clinical judgement (a biopsy may be performed to exclude a genuine skin condition). The lesions are difficult to treat until the underlying psychological condition improves. It is important for the doctor to maintain sympathetic contact, and to avoid confronting and alienating the patient. Psychotherapy or psychiatric referral may be indicated, as the condition may last for years.

DERMATITIS HERPETIFORMIS
A very itchy skin disease associated with coeliac disease affecting males more commonly than females.

The cause of this disease is unclear. It is found with coeliac disease (inability to absorb gluten from the intestine), although the sufferer may be unaware of any bowel problem when consulting the doctor about the rash. Small intensely itchy blisters are found on the elbows, knees, neck, shoulder and back, and a biopsy is required to confirm the diagnosis. Dapsone tablets may be prescribed initially to control symptoms, but all those affected should see a gastroenterologist for investigation into associated bowel problems, and a gluten-free diet should be commenced. Improvement is often rapid once treatment is started. The disease is controlled by a gluten-free diet, dapsone or both.

DERMATOFIBROMA
Benign nodules immediately beneath the skin surface.

This common condition is thought to be a local reaction to some form of injury, such as an insect bite, although the initial event may not be remembered. Dermatofibromas appear as firm nodules which usually cause no symptoms. They may be skin-coloured but are often darker. They are found most commonly in young female adults, particularly on the lower legs. A biopsy will be helpful to rule out anything more serious if the diagnosis is unclear. Irritating nodules can be removed under local anaesthetic, but since they are benign, no treatment may be necessary.

ECZEMA
Eczema and dermatitis are synonymous. The condition involves acute or subacute inflammation of the skin, centred in the epidermis and upper dermis.

Eczemas can be divided into exogenous (those caused by external factors) and endogenous (those related to a constitutional tendency to developing the eczema). The exogenous eczemas are contact irritant and contact allergic dermatitis (p. 138). The endogenous eczemas are atopic eczema, discoid eczema and pompholyx.

ATOPIC ECZEMA
Atopic eczema is the commonest eczema in childhood, affecting about 20 per cent of children in the UK. In the vast majority of patients it starts in childhood. Most do not have the condition as adults, but a few do have eczema through to adult life. Reactivation in adult life is often associated with work and is commonest in people who have to wash their skin frequently such as nurses, car mechanics and hairdressers. In infancy the eczema often

affects the face, in childhood it usually affects the skin creases in front of the elbows and behind the knees and in adult life focuses again on the face, and also on the hands.

The problem with the skin is threefold:
- The skin is dry and dry skin is irritable.
- Where the eczema develops the inflammation leads to further irritation.
- Scratching of irritated skin leads to loss of barrier function and allows infection to get in. Infection, particularly with *Staphylococcus aureus*, leads to worsening of the eczema, not only at the site that is infected but also at distant sites.

Atopic eczema is associated with asthma and hayfever and there is often a family history of asthma, eczema or hayfever. Treatment is with daily baths, avoidance of detergents, the use of emollients to wash the skin, copious moisturisers and appropriate strengths of topical corticosteroids, and topical and/or systemic antibiotics to treat infection.

Contact between patients with atopic eczema and those with cold sores must be avoided: the virus that causes cold sores can cause a widespread infection in the atopic individual which can spread to the blood and the brain.

DISCOID ECZEMA
This very aggressive eczema occurs usually in later life, in the 50s and 60s. The areas of eczema are round or coin shaped, well demarcated red areas that have a rough surface and are extremely itchy. Secondary infection is common. The disease is self-limiting and usually lasts for about 18 months. Treatment involves the use of emollients and moisturisers and relatively strong topical corticosteroids with antibiotics topically or systemically when infection occurs.

POMPHOLYX
Pompholyx is an acute or subacute eczema affecting the hands (cheiro-pompholyx) or the feet (pedo-pompholyx). Because the skin in these areas is very thick, the inflammation leads to accumulation of small collections of fluid allowing little vesicles – which look rather like sago grains in the skin – to develop. In the acute phase the skin is very itchy but as it goes through to a subacute and chronic phase the skin becomes thicker and drier so that fissures and splits can occur on the fingers and palms. Special care should be exercised in looking after the skin of affected areas. Affected persons should avoid contact with detergents, they should wear rubber gloves for wet work, but for no longer than 15 minutes at a time as this leads to sweating and softening of the skin. Rubber gloves should even be worn when washing hair as shampoo contains high

levels of detergent. Copious amounts of moisturiser and emollients should be used and strong topical corticosteroids are normally needed to control the disease. Secondary infection does occur and needs to be treated with antibiotics.

ERYTHEMA MULTIFORME
A toxic skin eruption triggered by several factors.

What are the causes?
The most common cause is herpes simplex infection (the virus that causes cold sores and genital herpes). Other viruses may be responsible, as can bacterial and fungal infections, drugs, pregnancy and malignant disease. In 50 per cent of cases no cause is identified.

What are the symptoms?
The typical pattern is eruption of red, circular, non-scaly plaques which clear from the centre to give typical 'target' lesions. The hands and feet are most commonly affected, but it can also occur in the mucous lining of the mouth and the eyes, a condition known as Steven Johnson syndrome. A severe variant exists, where the top layer of the skin is shed (known as toxic epidermal necrolysis). A biopsy can confirm the diagnosis.

What are the treatment options?
Identification and removal of the underlying cause is the mainstay of treatment. If large areas are affected oral steroids or hospital admission may be required. Individual lesions last a few days and several appear over 1–2 weeks until the underlying cause is removed.

ERYTHEMA NODOSUM
An inflammation of the subcutaneous fat.

This condition mostly affects young women and may be caused by a variety of infections or drug treatments, or it may indicate an underlying disease. In some cases no cause is found. Painful, dusky-red nodules, 1–5cm in diameter, are seen typically on the shins, sometimes with associated joint pains. Physical examination, chest X-ray and blood testing will help identify an underlying cause and a biopsy can be taken. Rest and anti-inflammatory drugs will relieve the pain. Any underlying cause should be treated. Individual lesions settle in 6–8 weeks, but the condition may persist if the cause is not found and removed.

FISH TANK GRANULOMA
A condition found in people who are involved in cleaning tropical fish tanks.

This condition is due to a mycobacterium which lives in fish tanks, and enters the skin through tiny breaks when the hands are in the water. These result in reddish-blue nodules, either singly or in groups, on the hands and forearms. The diagnosis is made on the appearance of the skin, and a biopsy can confirm this. Sick fish must be removed from the tank and gloves should be worn when cleaning it. Antibiotics can be used, as can steroid creams, but often avoiding bare hands in tank water is all that is necessary. Even after successful treatment, it may take months or years for the nodules to resolve.

FOLLICULITIS
Infection or inflammation of one or more hair follicles caused by bacterial or yeast infection.

Folliculitis is more common in overweight people and diabetics, and may be triggered by hair removal (by waxing or shaving, for example). Pustules appear in hair-bearing areas, often the beard area in men and the legs in women.
   Furuncles and carbuncles are related conditions where one or more hair follicles are infected forming an abscess.

What are the treatment options?
A microbiological swab can be taken to confirm the presence of infection and indicate the most appropriate treatment. Oral antibiotics and antibiotic cream are used to treat bacterial folliculitis. Yeast folliculitis responds to anti-fungal drugs. Folliculitis may be recurrent, in which case the use of antiseptic washes in the bath or shower can help keep infection at bay. Carbuncles may need to be drained.

FUNGAL INFECTIONS (RINGWORM)
These extremely common skin infections can affect several parts of the body.

Fungal infection can be contracted from other people or animals and affect the skin, hair and nails.

What are the symptoms?
These depend on the type and site of the infection. The most common type of ringworm (or tinea) is tinea pedis

(athlete's foot), which appears as scaly or soggy skin between the toes, especially the 4th and 5th toe. There may also be dry scaly skin on the feet with blistering.

Any area of skin can be involved in ringworm, with the rash appearing as red patches with a distinct, scaly edge (the 'ring') which is often itchy. Toenails are affected more commonly than fingernails. They become yellow, crumbly and thickened and may separate from the nail bed.

Ringworm affects the scalp in children more than adults, with scaly, coin-shaped areas of hair loss and scaly or boggy inflamed swelling with overlying hair loss (a kerion).

How is it diagnosed?
Diagnosis should be confirmed, particularly in nail infection, before treatment is started. Skin scrapings, nail clippings or hair pluckings are taken and sent for analysis.

What are the treatment options?
Antifungal creams are sufficient to clear up most skin infections, but if extensive, a course of oral treatment may be required. Antifungal nail lacquers are effective in some nail infections, but more commonly a 6–12 week course of tablets is needed. Scalp infection requires oral treatment. Treatment is generally effective but recurrence is common.

Steroids should be avoided: they cause the rash to worsen, and may change its appearance, making diagnosis difficult.

GRANULOMA ANNULARE
Lesions most commonly found on the hands and feet, although they can be more widespread.

The cause is not known, although widespread cases of granuloma annulare can be associated with diabetes. It commonly affects children and young adults, and is more often seen in females.

What are the symptoms?
The typical lesion consists of a clear centre surrounded by a collection of nodules forming a circle roughly 2cm in diameter. The nodules may be purple or skin-coloured.

What are the treatment options?
There is no truly effective treatment, but steroid creams or steroid injection into the affected area may be used. A urine sample should be tested for glucose to check for diabetes. Granuloma annulare resolves without treatment over several months to years, although recurrences are common.

HAIR LOSS
A common condition in both men and women, often known as alopecia.

What are the causes?
Generalised hair loss or thinning can have a variety of causes. The most common is androgenic alopecia, or male-pattern baldness, which can affect men from the teens. Half of women aged 50 are also affected to some extent, and the number increases with age in both sexes.

Abnormalities of the thyroid or pituitary glands, dietary deficiencies (p. 71) and certain medication, notably in chemotherapy, can lead to hair loss, which should be reversible on treating or removing the underlying cause.

Another cause is a condition known as telogen effluvium, where a large number of hairs are shed simultaneously, often about three months after an episode of physical or psychological stress (such as childbirth). This requires no treatment and reverts to normal in time.

What are the treatment options?
Most people with thinning hair require no treatment, and indeed treatment can be quite unsatisfactory. Lotions are available to apply to the scalp, and many patients derive some benefit from tablets. Private surgery in the form of hair transplant may be an option, and wigs can be prescribed by a hospital specialist.

Androgenic alopecia is progressive, although the degree of hair loss varies from one individual to another. If there is an underlying cause, hair loss is usually reversed when the cause is dealt with.

HEAD LICE
Infection with head lice is common, especially in primary school children, but any age can be affected.

What are the causes?
Head lice are not related to hygiene: they infect clean and dirty hair alike. The head louse cannot jump or fly, and spreads between people by walking across hair, so only close head-to-head contacts can be infected.

What are the symptoms?
Itching of the scalp and/or neck is the main symptom, and red spots are seen which may become infected with scabbing. Lice may be seen on the scalp. Empty egg cases are often seen attached to the base of hairs. These do not

indicate active infection. Insecticidal treatment is only indicated if live lice are present. The easiest way to check for live lice is by combing through sections of wet, conditioned hair. Wiping the comb on a tissue will reveal any lice present.

What are the treatment options?
A variety of preparations can be bought from the chemist, but it is best to avoid alcohol-based treatments which are highly inflammable, and can be irritant and trigger an asthma attack in susceptible individuals.

Head lice live for 30 days on the head, but only 24 hours off it. The female lays up to 100 eggs, which take 7–10 days to hatch; 10 days later a female can begin to lay eggs.

The preparation should be applied to clean, dry hair before going to bed, and left to dry naturally, washing out the next morning. This should be repeated after seven days. Empty egg cases are not removed by this treatment, and have to be physically removed by combing. An alternative treatment is the 'bug-busting' approach (p. 59). Kits are available from chemists and the treatment involves combing wet, conditioned hair every three days for at least two weeks.

Failure to check and treat close contacts is a common cause of re-infection. Two to three days after the second treatment, detection combing should be repeated. If treatment hasn't been successful, make an appointment with the GP, school nurse or health visitor for more advice.

HERPES SIMPLEX
The herpes simplex virus causes cold sores on the body and the genitals.

The condition consists of painful blisters which can ulcerate, and clear after 7–10 days. Attacks may be recurrent, and are contagious. Cold sores can be treated early with antiviral cream, which should be applied as soon as tingling is felt, before the blisters appear. Genital herpes can be treated with antiviral tablets and condoms should be used to protect sexual partners from infection.

HIDRADENITIS SUPPURITIVA
Hidradenitis is a disorder of the apocrine glands of the skin, affecting approximately 1 in 500 people.

What are the symptoms?
The condition starts usually between the ages of 20 and 30 and is more common in females. Painful, inflamed nodules and abscesses are seen in the groin, armpits and sometimes the neck, often with blackheads which may leave scarring. Sufferers have 4–5 new boils a month in typical sites, each of which may be sore for about 7 days. Stress, heat, sweating and friction tend to make it worse and it is more common in smokers.

What are the treatment options?
Antiseptic washes and antibiotic creams may be enough in mild cases but often long-term courses of antibiotics (lasting at least three months) are necessary. In women, a type of contraceptive pill can be useful.

In severe cases with multiple lesions, steroid tablets may be used for a few days, and isotretinoin – available from hospital dermatologists – can also help. It is an effective treatment, but can cause fetal abnormalities if taken in pregnancy, so care has to be taken before initiating this treatment. Surgery can be used for acute abscesses.

What is the outlook?
Hidradenitis often runs a prolonged course, and may be present for up to 20 years after diagnosis. It may settle in women after the menopause, due to hormonal changes.

HIRSUTISM
Hirsutism describes the growth of hair in a male pattern on the body and face of a female.

What are the causes?
In most cases, no cause is found, and it is simply due to an increased sensitivity to male hormones which are normally found in the female circulation. Polycystic ovarian syndrome is a known cause, while abnormalities of the pituitary or adrenal glands are less common causes.

What are the symptoms?
Excess hair is seen mainly down the midline of the body – lips, chin, sternum and abdomen. Menstrual irregularities may be present, and the skin may be greasy. A blood test can confirm an underlying ovarian or gland problem while polycystic ovaries will be visible on an ultrasound scan.

What are the treatment options?
Any underlying medical condition should be treated. Bleaching can be tried or hair removal by plucking or shaving. A beautician can advise on waxing or electrolysis, and laser hair removal is available in some hospitals. A form

of the oral contraceptive pill is used in polycystic ovarian syndrome, to counteract the male hormones and to regularise periods. Patients who are overweight often benefit from a weight loss programme.

In cases where no cause is found, symptoms tend to start at puberty and may worsen with age.

HYPERHIDROSIS
Hyperhidrosis is an excess production of sweat.

What are the causes?
Excess sweat production may be localised to the palms, soles and armpits, or generalised over the whole body. It may be due to heat, emotion, medicines, shock, or a disorder of the glands or nerves controlling sweating. Generalised increased sweating is more likely if an underlying cause is present; blood tests and/or X-rays may be performed if an underlying condition is suspected.

What are the treatment options?
Aluminium chloride-based antiperspirant lotions can be applied in affected areas – these are available from a doctor and may be all that is required.

For stubborn cases, a process called iontophoresis can be performed in hospital clinics. This involves the passage of a low voltage electrical current across the skin. Several treatments are required, and the course may need to be repeated or continued to keep symptoms under control.

Surgery is required in some cases to interrupt the nerves which supply the sweat glands. A new approach is the use of Botox injections into the affected areas of skin.

ICHTHYOSIS
A condition resulting in a scale-like appearance of the skin; the term is derived from the Greek for fish.

What are the causes?
A combination of increased production of skin cells and altered adhesion between cells, causes dead cells or 'scales' to remain stuck to the skin surface. Ichthyosis may be inherited, although the condition can develop later in life.

What are the symptoms?
The most common form of ichthyosis, ichthyosis vulgaris, affects 1 person in 300 and first appears in infancy. Persistent mild scaling of the back, abdomen, thighs and upper arms is seen, which worsens in winter. Another form, recessive ichthyosis, is carried on the X chromosome and affects males only, causing large, dark scales on the neck, buttocks, trunk and limbs. Female carriers of the condition can suffer prolonged labour due to the lack of the enzyme steroid sulphatase. The condition does not tend to improve with age. More severe inherited forms exist, which are generally evident from birth.

The development of acquired ichthyosis later in life is unusual, and may indicate underlying illness. It is important to differentiate between this and normal drying of the skin found later in life.

What are the treatment options?
Emollients, both as soap substitutes and moisturisers, are the mainstay of treatment, combined with gentle abrasion to remove the scales. Creams containing weak concentrations of salicylic acid can dissolve the scales, but care must be taken on broken skin and in infants as absorption can lead to internal organ damage. Tablet treatment is sometimes used under specialist supervision in severe cases.

For more severe types of inherited ichthyosis, genetic intervention may be a treatment of the future.

IMPETIGO
A bacterial infection characterised by 'weeping' blisters.

What are the symptoms?
Small blisters appear on a background of red skin. These burst, releasing pus which dries to give honey-coloured crusts. Local lymph nodes may be enlarged and tender. It is most often seen on the exposed skin of children, and is very contagious in this age group. The presence of infection can be confirmed by the GP taking a swab.

What are the treatment options?
Affected children should be kept off school until the area starts to heal, and towels should not be shared. Very mild cases may settle simply with regular cleaning. If a few small areas are affected, antibiotic cream should be used for 7–10 days. For more extensive cases, oral antibiotics are used in combination with cream for a seven-day period.

Most episodes will settle with the above measures. If not, a swab is necessary to check for unusual bacteria, and the possibility of re-infection from an untreated source should be considered. Impetigo may develop into the more severe condition of cellulitis (p. 137) if not treated effectively.

ITCH
Itch is the most common symptom of skin disease.

The term 'itch' is used to describe the sensation which makes us want to scratch. The mechanism of itch is poorly understood, and a variety of chemicals are thought to be involved. One of the most important is histamine, which is contained in mast cells found in the skin. Antihistamines are used to relieve itch in skin conditions like eczema.

Expectation plays a part in itch. Hearing someone talk about bugs and insects, for example, can set off a desire to scratch, even though there is no actual physical stimulation of the skin. Itch may also be caused by diseases of the skin or the internal organs, as a side-effect of drugs or due to excessive drying of the skin.

There is no specific cure for itch. Scratching is thought to relieve itch by sending a stronger signal to the brain, thus overwhelming the weaker impulse which caused the itch.

KELOID
Keloid scarring is an exaggerated or overgrown response to injury, although it may also occur spontaneously in undamaged skin.

What are the symptoms?
Raised reddish purple or flesh-coloured scars, which may extend beyond the boundaries of the original wound are typical. Keloids are most often seen on the chest, neck, back and shoulders, especially in young adults, although they can appear in older people. They are also more prevalent in people of Afro-Caribbean origin. It is thought that there is an inherited tendency to develop this type of scarring.

What are the treatment options?
Steroids can be used to try to reduce the scars. Steroid cream applied regularly may help, but more often steroid injected into the keloid is required – small amounts of steroid are injected into the surface of the affected skin. Over repeated injections the colouring and bulk of the scar may reduce, giving a more acceptable cosmetic appearance. Steroid-impregnated tape can also be applied, which is available through GPs.

What is the outlook?
After one episode of keloid scarring, it is likely that the problem will recur with future skin damage. Unnecessary operations and procedures should therefore be avoided.

KERATOACANTHOMA
A benign growth found in sun-exposed parts of the body, particularly in fair-skinned individuals.

What are the symptoms?
A small papule appears suddenly and grows quite quickly over a matter of weeks to produce a large nodule, 1–2cm in diameter, with a horny plug in the centre.

What are the treatment options?
If keratoacanthomas are left, they will naturally resolve without any treatment, but this will leave a noticeable scar. Also, it can be difficult to differentiate keratoacanthomas from certain types of skin cancer. Because of this, they are removed under local anaesthetic. Once removed, it is unlikely there will be problems.

KERATOSIS PILARIS
Patches of rough skin.

What are the symptoms?
This is an inherited condition which begins in childhood. Hair follicles fill with horny plugs of dead skin cells leaving rough skin, often with small red or greyish papules around the hair follicles. The outer thighs and upper arms are most commonly involved but the face may also be affected.

What are the treatment options?
General measures such as the use of emollient soap substitutes, avoiding showers/baths that are too hot and patting rather than rubbing the skin dry may be helpful. Emollients should be used regularly to moisturise the skin, and those containing urea are particularly recommended. The condition generally becomes less obvious in adult life.

LEG ULCERS
Skin loss developing in discoloured or swollen skin.

What are the causes?
Venous leg ulcers are caused by impaired drainage of blood away from the leg and back to the heart. Arterial ulcers are due to impaired circulation causing a reduced amount of blood to reach the leg. Ulcers can also be caused by inflammation in the walls of the blood vessels (vasculitis).

The most common types of leg ulcer are venous (70 per cent), arterial (10 per cent) and those due to diabetes (5 per cent).

What are the symptoms?

Venous ulcers are usually preceded by a heaviness and swelling of the lower leg, which may last for years. The skin can become discoloured (red/brown) due to leakage of blood from the damaged blood vessels and there may be eczema in affected areas. Ulceration is most common around the ankle bones, and ulcers may be single or multiple and vary in size and depth.

Arterial ulcers are more commonly found on the toes, heel or front of the foot. There may be other evidence of arterial problems such as angina, or calf pain on walking.

Vasculitic ulcers start as painful spots, becoming small 'punched out' ulcers.

How is it diagnosed?

Blood tests including a diabetes check may be performed. Swabs may be taken if infection is suspected. The circulation should be tested to determine the type of ulcer and therefore the most appropriate treatment.

What are the treatment options?

Rest and elevation of the leg are important parts of the treatment for venous ulceration. The main aim is to relieve the swelling and pressure bandaging is very effective (although not to be used in arterial ulceration as this may worsen the circulation further). The bandages may be changed several times a week depending on the state of the ulcer. Any infection is treated with antibiotic cream or tablets. Varicose vein surgery may help by improving the venous drainage of the leg. For arterial ulcers, surgery may be necessary to improve the circulation. In vasculitic ulcers, the aim is to treat the underlying cause.

What is the outlook?

Healing is a slow process and can take years; some ulcers never heal. Once varicose ulcers have healed, compression stockings should be worn daily to try to prevent recurrence.

LEPROSY

Also known as Hansen's disease, after the Norwegian doctor who discovered the responsible bacteria.

Leprosy is due to infection with a similar type of bacterium to that which causes tuberculosis. It is spread by droplet infection and close contact, much like flu, and although not found naturally in Britain, it remains an important problem in parts of Asia and Africa. Well-defined areas of altered

---

AT THE LEADING EDGE

The eradication of leprosy

In 1991 the World Health Organization launched its target of eliminating leprosy as a global health problem by 2000 through:

- Ensuring all health centres had adequate stocks of multidrug treatment (MDT).
- Education campaigns to encourage people with 'suspicious' skin markings to seek treatment.
- Health education to ensure patients took all medications regularly and completely.
- Keeping accurate records to monitor progress.

Elimination was defined as less than one new case per 10,000 population and the target was met. Despite the global reduction in cases, however, leprosy remains a significant problem in six countries: Brazil, Madagascar, India, Myanmar, Nepal and Mozambique. Efforts are now being aimed at reducing the prevalence of the disease in those countries, and repeating the global success at the local level in those areas and regions where leprosy is still common – largely sub-Saharan and central Africa and Indonesia.

---

pigment are seen, which are numb, leading to an increased risk of injury. There may be ulceration of the skin, and some areas become thickened, particularly on the face. A biopsy of the skin and nerves confirms the diagnosis. Treatment – in the form of dapsone in combination with oral antituberculous drugs – may be required for life.

LICHEN PLANUS

A common, sometimes chronic, skin disorder.

Most common in middle age, males and females are affected equally by this condition. Shiny, purple, flat-topped papules are found on the skin in varying sizes, often with clusters round the wrists, ankles and genitalia. The papules can also be seen in areas of skin damage (the appearance of a skin condition in areas of broken or damaged skin is known as the Koebner phenomenon). The lesions are often itchy, although may cause no symptoms. In 50 per cent of cases, the mucous membranes are involved (lining of the mouth, genital area) and these areas may be affected alone. In 10 per cent of cases the fingernails are affected, causing grooving and ridging of the nail. A similar appearance can be caused by some prescribed drugs, so a skin biopsy may be performed to confirm the diagnosis.

What are the treatment options?

Treatment can only control symptoms – it is not curative, and takes the form of steroid cream or ointment applied twice daily when itchy. If the condition is very severe or widespread, steroid tablets may be prescribed and a steroid paste or spray can be used for painful mouth lesions.

Lichen planus tends to settle on its own over a period of three months to two years, although affected areas may appear darker than usual for some months afterwards (this is known as post-inflammatory hyperpigmentation). If the mouth is affected, this can take decades to resolve, and there is a very small risk of developing localised skin cancer within the mouth. Phototherapy (p. 112) may be used for stubborn itch. Less than 20 per cent of sufferers will have a further attack in their lifetime.

LICHEN SCLEROSUS ET ATROPHICUS
An inflammatory disease mainly affecting middle-aged to elderly women, although it may occur in children.

What are the symptoms?
This condition usually targets the genital area, causing itch, painful intercourse, and pain on passing urine, although it may be asymptomatic. The skin of the labia and clitoris appears white, shiny and thinning, and there may be loss of the normal structure in more advanced cases. It can less commonly affect skin at virtually any other body site. There is a male equivalent, involving the penis, known as balanitis xerotica obliterans.

How is it diagnosed?
Diagnosis is generally made by appearance, although a biopsy can be helpful, and is essential in areas not responding to treatment. Other conditions such as allergic skin disease may need to be excluded.

What are the treatment options?
Treatment consists of using a soap substitute for washing, combined with a strong steroid cream regularly initially, then used as needed. In advanced cases, removal of the foreskin in men will take out affected skin; surgery in women and children is an option once the condition is under control and scarred or damaged skin can be excised.

This condition can progress to skin cancer, although this is rare and can take many years. It is important to notify a GP of any areas that are changing or unresponsive to treatment.

LICHEN SIMPLEX
Also known as neurodermatitis, this skin problem is partly self inflicted.

Lichen simplex is caused by repeated rubbing or scratching to a certain area of skin, either out of habit or as a manifestation of stress. There is not necessarily any underlying skin complaint. The skin becomes red and thickened with obvious creases. The back of the neck, lower legs, and ano-genital area are common sites to be affected and biopsy is only necessary if the diagnosis is in doubt. Steroid creams combined with covering of the affected area may help to break the habit and affected sites will settle with treatment. However, patches do tend to recur either in the same site or elsewhere.

LUPUS ERYTHEMATOSUS
A multisystem autoimmune disorder which may be limited in some cases to the skin.

What are the causes?
Lupus is caused by the body producing antibodies against itself. It may affect the skin alone, or other body systems too. Any internal organ may be affected. It is more common in females, and in the black and Chinese populations.

What are the symptoms?
The rash seen in lupus consists of scaly red plaques, often in sun-exposed sites, although any area may be affected. A redness of the cheeks and nose is common. The lesions may settle to leave scarring, and alopecia may be a feature.

How is it diagnosed?
No single test exists to diagnose lupus. If it is suspected, blood and urine testing, plus a skin biopsy are necessary to determine the type and extent of involvement.

What are the treatment options?
Sunlight aggravates the skin condition in lupus in 25 per cent of patients, and should be avoided with the use of high-factor sunscreen and sun-protective clothing. Strong steroid creams are used on the rash and these may be combined

with steroid tablets in more severe cases. Anti-malarial drugs are helpful in extensive cases, and these, along with other treatments, may be prescribed by a hospital specialist.

There is no cure for lupus; the aim is to control symptoms. Many cases of skin-restricted lupus resolve spontaneously.

LYME DISEASE
Named after Lyme, Connecticut, where the disease was first recognised, this condition results from a tick bite.

This condition is caused by the microorganism *Borrelia burgdorferi*, which is transmitted by the bite of a tick. Not everyone affected recalls being bitten, but after about a week, a slowly expanding red circular patch forms around the bite. In some cases, the infection may spread to other areas of the body, and may cause joint pains, irregularities of the heartbeat, and nervous system problems. Diagnosis can be confirmed by a blood test. If only the skin is involved, oral antibiotics are used; intravenous antibiotics are necessary if any spread of infection has occurred. Antibiotics should cure the skin infection. However, if the disease has spread, cure is not always guaranteed even with intensive treatment.

MALIGNANT MELANOMA
The least common, but potentially fatal, skin cancer.

What are the causes?
Sunburn, particularly in childhood, plays a major role in the development of this cancer. Having an immediate family member who has had melanoma increases the risk, as does the presence of multiple moles. Females are more commonly affected than males, and the incidence is rapidly increasing.

What are the symptoms?
Although melanomas often occur in normal skin, when they appear like a 'new' mole, one in three arises in an existing mole. Any of the following changes in a mole should be checked:

Scotland has the highest UK rate of malignant melanoma. Researchers are unsure whether this is due to the higher numbers of people with Celtic (fair-skinned) colouring.

- asymmetry;
- border irregularity;
- colour irregularity.

Other changes to note are inflammation, crusting, itching or bleeding. A mole on any part of the body can be affected, including fingernails, toenails and soles.

How is it diagnosed?
A full examination is necessary. If melanoma is suspected, the affected area should be removed. Blood tests and X-rays may be performed, depending on the extent of the tumour. Chemotherapy, radiotherapy, surgery or immunotherapy may be used in more advanced cases.

What is the outlook?
The prognosis depends on the thickness of the melanoma; for thin melanomas the outlook is excellent. Diagnosis at an early stage is therefore important. Regular follow-up appointments are essential after removal to check the original site and the rest of the skin for suspicious areas.

MILIA
Milia – tiny white spots on the skin – are very common.

Milia may occur on areas of damaged skin, or in sweat ducts or sebaceous glands as white cysts, especially on the face. They occur at any age and are commonest in young women. No treatment is necessary but the overlying skin can be pierced with the tip of a sterile needle and the cyst removed, if wished. Milia are likely to go away without treatment, although many are removed for cosmetic reasons.

MOLES AND PIGMENTATION
Areas of pigmented and often raised skin.

The average white-skinned adult may have up to 50 moles. The presence of more than this number is a risk factor for developing malignant melanoma, so individuals with a large number should cover up and take extra care in the sun.

ACQUIRED MELANOCYTIC NAEVUS
This is the most common type of mole, which is roughly 2–3mm in diameter, with a regular colour. These usually appear from early childhood. No treatment is required unless there is concern about possible malignant change, in which case they can be surgically removed.

ATYPICAL NAEVI
These may have an irregular edge or colour, or may be inflamed. Increased numbers may be found in people with melanoma. Suspicious examples should be removed. If present in large numbers, the doctor will usually recommend referral to hospital for regular photography and monitoring.

CHLOASMA/ MELASMA

This is an increase in pigment production due to hormonal changes and is commonly seen on the faces of pregnant women or those on the contraceptive pill. Sunlight darkens the pigment, so use of a sunscreen is recommended.

CONGENITAL NAEVI

These are present from birth and found in about 1 per cent of all babies. They can vary in size from a few millimetres to covering a large area of the body although this is rare.

FRECKLES

Freckles are due to an increased production of pigment in localised areas in the skin. These are stimulated by the sun to give the very common flat light-brown macules. They are especially common in fair-haired people and red-heads, and indicate a sensitivity to the sun.

HALO NAEVUS

This is seen most commonly on the backs of teenagers, and is so called because there is a circle of paler skin around the mole, which will often fade completely. This is due to immunological attack on the mole which is destroyed, with some loss of surrounding pigment cells. The pale skin is prone to burning so should be protected in the sun.

LIVER SPOTS

These flat brown macules are common on sun-exposed sites from middle age. They have a regular colour and distinct edge and may be treated with cryotherapy (p. 119). Malignant change is possible over many years, so any change in colour or size should be reported to your doctor.

MOLLUSCUM CONTAGIOSUM

Small skin lesions, commonly seen in children.

This is due to viral infection, and affects mainly children. It is spread by direct contact, through sharing towels for example, with shiny whitish-pink nodules with a small pit in the centre appearing 2–6 weeks after contact. They can affect any area of the body. Multiple lesions are common, and they may be particularly numerous in children with eczema. Although generally without symptoms, they can become inflamed. An iodine-based paint can be prescribed for inflamed areas (but this is not commonly used); generally the condition resolves without treatment. Recovery may take up to 18 months and the condition does not recur.

MYCOSIS FUNGOIDES

A low-grade cancer of the immune system, which also involves the skin.

What are the symptoms?

Mycosis fungoides affects less than 1 in 100,000 of the population, commonly middle-aged adults. Its cause is unknown, although genetic, environmental and viral triggers may all play a part. Red scaly patches, especially in covered sites such as the buttocks, trunk, upper inner arms and thighs appear. This progresses to plaques, then skin tumours, and may eventually affect other systems in the body. The whole process may take many years. The patches may be itchy or asymptomatic. It can be difficult to differentiate between the early lesions and the much more common conditions of eczema and psoriasis. In the later stages, hair loss and enlarged lymph nodes may be present.

How is it diagnosed?

Diagnosis is made by skin biopsy, although this can be inconclusive in the early stages and may need to be repeated over a number of years. In later stages, blood tests can help to indicate if spread to other areas has taken place.

What are the treatment options?

Follow-up is necessary to assess the stage and to look for evidence of internal spread. In the pre-cancerous stages, symptoms may be controlled by the regular use of emollients and topical steroids. Phototherapy (p. 112) can relieve symptoms and also lead to remission. However, the majority of cases relapse when treatment stops. Radiotherapy and /or chemotherapy is used in later stages.

What is the outlook?

The outlook can be good: most individuals with the condition die in old age from other causes. In a few cases, however, advanced disease may be reached in two to three years.

NAPPY RASH

A raw, often blistering rash on a baby's skin.

What are the causes?

The most common cause of nappy rash is irritation from prolonged contact with urine and faeces, although the occurrence of nappy rash is reducing due to the increased use of absorbent disposable nappies. Nappy rash can also be due to infection with candida (the organism which causes thrush) and may be one of the areas affected by seborrhoeic dermatitis (p. 153). Psoriasis is a rare cause of nappy rash, as is eczema.

What are the symptoms?
The skin becomes red, inflamed and sore and there may be blistering and ulceration in more severe cases. In simple cases of irritant nappy rash, the skin folds in the groin tend to be spared, but are involved in candidal and seborrhoeic cases. In candidal nappy rash, small satellite spots may be seen separate from the main area of redness.

What are the treatment options?
Nappies should be changed frequently. At each change, the nappy area should be cleaned thoroughly with a soap substitute or simply water. Liberal amounts of barrier cream, such as petroleum jelly, should then be applied. Baby wipes may contain fragrance which can irritate broken skin, so these should not be used. Nappies should be left off for short periods. In candidal infection or seborrhoeic dermatitis, a steroid cream combined with an antifungal agent may help.

NECROBIOSIS LIPOIDICA
Painless plaques on the fronts of the shins.

Necrobiosis lipoidica is associated with diabetes, although less than 1 per cent of diabetics are affected. It also appears in non-diabetics, or before diabetes has been diagnosed. It is characterised by shiny, waxy yellow/red plaques with easily visible blood vessels. These are not usually sore or itchy, but may ulcerate and be difficult to heal. Diagnosis is made on appearance, although biopsy can be helpful if there is any doubt. Diabetes should be tested for if not already known to be present. This condition is typically persistent and difficult to treat, although steroid creams may be tried, and cosmetics can be used to cover the affected areas.

NEUROFIBROMATOSIS
Multiple abnormalities of soft tissue and nerves.

What are the causes?
This genetically determined disease affects 1 in 3000 of the population, although 50 per cent have no affected family member and the cause is a new gene mutation. There are two types: type 1 is known as Von Recklinghausen's disease and affects the skin; type 2 affects the nervous system.

What are the symptoms?
Multiple neurofibromas are seen. These are soft, flesh-coloured, dome-shaped nodules a few millimetres to several centimetres in diameter. Typically they feel as if they can be pushed inwards, as if through a buttonhole. Other features include the presence of freckles in the axillary (armpit) area, and at least six light brown patches (known as café-au-lait patches) appear before one year of age. However, neurofibromas tend not to be seen until puberty and increase in number throughout life.

What are the treatment options?
If neurofibromatosis is suspected, hospital referral is needed for confirmation and further management. Large neurofibromas can be removed if a nuisance. Hospital follow-up is recommended, and confirmed cases should receive genetic counselling regarding future family.

What is the outlook?
There is a small risk of neurofibromas becoming malignant. In the future, DNA screening prior to conception may help to identify those at risk. Children of affected adults have a 1 in 2 chance of developing the disease.

PAPULAR URTICARIA
The manifestation of an allergic reaction to insect bites.

Itchy papules – especially on the arms and legs, but often distributed asymmetrically across the body – tend to occur in groups and settle leaving a small scar or area of increased colouring. The spots can become infected due to scratching. Diagnosis is usually made on examination. It can be confirmed by identifying the cause. Pets should be examined by a vet. Grooming pets over a polythene sheet will catch any bugs they may be harbouring, and these can then be taken to the vet for analysis.

Anti-itch creams or calamine lotion can be used to relieve the symptoms, as can antihistamines, but the main treatment is to eradicate the cause: insect repellents may be needed.

PARONYCHIA
An infection in the skin surrounding the fingernails and toenails.

Paronychia may be acute – lasting a few days or so – caused by bacteria entering through damaged skin or the cuticle. The nail fold is tender and swollen and pus may be produced. There is also a chronic version which may be due to a combination of bacteria and/or yeast organisms. In chronic paronychia the nail can be ridged and discoloured. Chronic paronychia is more common in people with diabetes, with poor circulation, recurrent vaginal thrush, and in those who do wet work, or work with flour.

Any pus produced should be swabbed and tested. Testing for diabetes and vaginal thrush may be necessary. Oral antibiotics or antifungals in combination with antifungal cream are used depending on the identified cause. Over-manicuring of the cuticles should be stopped, and the hands should be kept warm and dry. Acute paronychias generally settle with antibiotics, although occasionally they need to be lanced to release a build-up of pus.

PEMPHIGOID/PEMPHIGUS
Conditions in which the skin blisters and separates.

These two conditions are autoimmune disorders: antibodies are produced by the body which attack some of the proteins that hold the layers of the skin together, leading to separation and blister formation. In pemphigus the blisters form near the skin surface; in pemphigoid the problem is deeper.

Pemiphigoid tends to affect the elderly. Blisters may arise anywhere and can be very itchy. Pemphigus sufferers tend to be younger and may be more unwell. It is a severe condition – potentially fatal in extreme cases. Blisters may appear first in the mouth, making eating painful, and spread to the face, back, chest and scalp. The blisters rupture easily.

Diagnosis is confirmed by biopsy, and blood tests may be performed to test for antibodies in the circulation. Strong steroid creams are used in combination with steroid tablets. In pemphigus, hospital admission may be necessary. Steroids may be required for several months in a gradually reducing dose. However, the natural progression is for these conditions to burn out over a period of months to years.

PILONIDAL SINUS
A condition in which one or more hairs ingrow into the skin of the cleft of the buttocks, causing inflammation and often leading to abscess formation.

The condition affects more men than women and is rare after the age of 40. It can cause and may produce a discharge. Antibiotics may be of some benefit, but often

surgery to remove the hair, drain the abscess, then close the skin is the only effective treatment. This can often be treated as a day case, under sedation and local anaesthetic.

PITYRIASIS ROSEA
An often otherwise asymptomatic red rash.

Pityriasis rosea is most common in young adults and children, especially in the spring and autumn. It starts as a single, 2–4cm diameter red patch, which is followed about a week later by crops of similar lesions with a fine scale on the chest, abdomen, back and upper arms. The lesions on the back may be lined up along the skin creases giving a 'Christmas tree' appearance. The rash is usually asymptomatic but may be itchy. Although the cause has not been confirmed it may be viral. It is not caused by a fungus or bacteria, nor is it due to an allergy.

Like some viral diseases, pityriasis rosea usually occurs only once. Unlike many viruses, however, pityriasis rosea does not seem to be contagious.

This condition is benign and usually resolves in 4–8 weeks, with no recurrence. Moisturisers and anti-itch creams may be used if necessary. Sunlight may hasten recovery.

PITYRIASIS VERSICOLOR
A mild fungal infection causing changes in pigment.

This non-infectious condition is caused by overgrowth of yeasts, which normally live on the skin, in response to hot, humid conditions. Acids released by the yeasts cause alteration in skin pigmentation. Young adults are most commonly affected, with pale brown or pinkish oval papules appearing on the trunk. In the sun these areas do not tan.

Skin scrapings reveal the responsible yeasts. Antifungal creams can be applied at night for several weeks, in combination with the use of antifungal shampoo twice a week, using the lather to wash the body. Oral antifungal tablets may also be taken. Untreated areas will persist, but treated areas will return to normal. Recurrences are common.

POLYMORPHIC LIGHT ERUPTION
A condition that results from being in the sun.

Itchy red plaques, papules and vesicles appear in exposed areas within 24 hours of sun exposure. Females are more commonly affected and there may be a history of the condition in the family. The rash appears in spring and persists through the summer but improves as a tan develops. It tends to recur annually.

The regular use of sunscreen and sun-protective clothing may be sufficient to control the condition in mild cases. Weak steroid cream can be used to settle the rash. Desensitisation treatment is commonly used: a short course of phototherapy (p. 112) is given in the spring to 'harden' the skin to the effects of the sun, and give a mild protective tan. Light testing can be performed in hospitals to look for an exaggerated response to controlled amounts.

PORPHYRIA
A multisystem metabolic disorder, which in the past may have triggered some of the myths surrounding werewolves, as its symptoms include a low tolerance of sunlight and excessive growth of body hair.

The porphyrias are a group of rare, inherited disorders in which an enzyme is lacking, leading to a build-up of proteins in the bloodstream. These proteins, known as porphyrins, are toxic to the nervous system and cause increased sensitivity to sunlight. The skin becomes fragile and may develop red blisters, especially on the face and back of the hands. Scarring and increased hair growth may occur in these sites.

Porphyrins can be tested for by a hospital specialist. The porphyrin level is treated and kept down by regular removal of a proportion of the blood from the circulation. Sunscreens are necessary, and anti-malarial drugs may be helpful. There is no cure at present for some of the porphyrias, although in time gene therapy may be possible. However, some types may be cured simply by removal of triggering factors, such as alcohol and some medications.

PSORIASIS
A chronic scaling skin disorder, often hereditary.

What are the causes?
The cause of psoriasis is not completely understood, but there is a hereditary component, with 80 per cent of psoriasis due to genetic factors. The underlying problem is a more rapid life cycle of the cells which make up the epidermis. Psoriasis may be triggered in susceptible individuals by factors such as infection or drugs (such as beta-blockers); it is then made worse by factors such as stress or alcohol.

What are the symptoms?
Psoriasis may develop at any age. It typically consists of well-demarcated red plaques with a silvery scaly surface. The knees and elbows are common sites but any area may be affected. The scalp is often involved, with thick scales, and the nails may have multiple small pits. Scars or areas of injury tend to be a focus for psoriasis (known as the Koebner phenomenon), and arthritis may also be a feature.

There are 1.5 million people with psoriasis in the UK. It is rare under the age of 10, but may start in the teens, 20s or 30s. Some people first show symptoms in retirement.

Guttate psoriasis is a particular type seen following throat infections in children and young adults. The psoriasis plaques are smaller (like rain drops) and tend to resolve with no treatment within about two months. A minority of sufferers may go on to develop psoriasis in adult life.

How is it diagnosed?
Diagnosis is made on the appearance of the condition. Skin lesions and nails may be mistaken for fungal infection, in which case skin scrapings and nail clippings will be analysed.

What are the treatment options?
There is no cure for psoriasis; the aim of treatment is to control and suppress symptoms and try to delay flare-ups.

Moisturisers should be used to reduce scale. A variety of creams including coal tar, steroids and vitamin D based creams can be used on the plaques. Coal tar can be messy, but the newer preparations are easier and cleaner to use. Strong steroids, although effective, may cause a rebound worsening when stopped. Vitamin D based creams increase maturation of the cells and modulate the immune response causing the disorder, and should be the treatment of choice. They may be used with steroids to counteract inflammation.

Sunlight or phototherapy (p. 112) is an effective treatment for most people and may provide relief for several months or longer. For severe cases, cytotoxic tablets may be prescribed, although these all have potential side effects, so regular blood tests are necessary. Shampoos are available for scalp psoriasis, and if necessary the scale can be softened with olive oil or proprietary creams prior to shampooing out. Nail psoriasis is hard to treat, but may improve with oral treatments. These are, however, not usually recommended.

What is the outlook?
Psoriasis is a life-long condition, but it is possible to go for long periods with no symptoms. It is important not to let the treatment become more of a nuisance than the condition.

If one parent has psoriasis, their child has a 25–30 per cent chance of having the condition. This goes up to 60 per cent if both parents are affected.

PYODERMA GANGRENOSUM
Ulcers caused by rapid inflammation of the skin.

This is often found in conjunction with other conditions, such as inflammatory bowel disease, arthritis or vasculitis (p. 152). The cause is not fully understood, but it may be due to an abnormal reaction by the immune system. Ulcers develop either singly or in crops, most commonly on the lower legs. These may start as a pustule or nodule with surrounding redness, which rapidly extends to give an ulcer with a distinct, reddish-purple edge. They are painful and there may be associated fever, with general aches and pains. Diagnosis is made on appearance and biopsy. Depending on other symptoms, further tests may be needed to look for associated conditions. The ulcers will require a dressing, with rest and elevation to encourage healing. Oral steroids are used to control the condition and prevent further spread. It may take months for pyoderma gangrenosum to clear, but treatment of any associated condition may hasten recovery.

PYOGENIC GRANULOMA
A small fleshy vascular nodule formed in response to trauma, commonly on the hands or feet.

Pyogenic granulomas develop within days or weeks in sites of trauma, such as a prick by a needle or thorn, although the incident is not always remembered. The surface of the nodule is fragile and tends to bleed easily when knocked. Diagnosis is usually clear to a doctor from appearance. However, as certain skin cancers can share this appearance, the removed tissue is always analysed. The nodule may reduce without treatment, but due to inconvenience and bleeding, surgical removal may be recommended.

ROSACEA
A disorder causing chronic inflammation of the face.

What are the causes?
The cause is unknown, but inherited susceptibility is likely to play a part. Demodex mites, which are naturally present in hair follicles and associated sebaceous glands, are found in larger numbers in rosacea sufferers but it is unlikely they are involved in its evolution. Certain foodstuffs such as tea, coffee, chocolate, cheese, alcohol, curries, vinegar and citrus fruits may aggravate the condition but patients should never be put on an exclusion diet without identifying the exacerbating agents for themselves. It can also be worsened by sun, wind, cold, heat and cigarette smoke. Steroid creams and ointments can also exacerbate it.

What are the symptoms?
Rosacea affects approximately 1 per cent of 30–60 year olds, although it may be seen from the early teens. Women are commonly affected, although it is often more severe in men.

In the early stages, flushing (which is more intense than normal blushing) is the most common feature. The flushing episodes become more prolonged, until a fixed redness of the face develops, affecting the nose, cheeks, chin and forehead. Papules and pustules then develop in the sites of redness, and in more severe cases the skin can become unevenly thickened (in rhinophyma, swelling of the nose, for example, which may be mistaken as being related to alcohol). The skin is typically more irritable and sensitive, and in 50 per cent of sufferers, the eyes will also be affected (ocular rosacea). The diagnosis is generally made on clinical appearance and history.

What are the treatment options?
There is no cure for rosacea, but in most patients it is self-limiting. A variety of treatments can be used to control the symptoms. The use of oil-free and fragrance-free skincare products is beneficial, and a soap substitute is less irritating for washing. Green-tinted foundation can counteract the red appearance. The avoidance of triggering factors, and regular use of a sunscreen (at least factor 20) can also help.

If these simple measures are not sufficient, antibiotic gels or creams can be prescribed if necessary in combination with antibiotic tablets. Antibiotics are taken in full dose for 2–3 weeks, then reduced according to symptoms. Flushing or redness can be treated using drugs with specific effects on blood vessels. With successful treatment, the papules and pustules tend to reduce first, but the reddening takes longer to respond. Antibiotic treatment may be required for months or years. Severe cases of rosacea may need referral to a hospital specialist for alternative treatments, including surgery for rhinophyma and laser treatment to reduce facial redness.

Although the condition does tend to resolve in time, it may persist for anything from a year to several decades.

SCABIES
The skin's response to infestation by a mite.

What are the causes?
Scabies is caused by the mite *Sarcoptes scabei*. It is transferred from person to person through close body contact, although 4–6 weeks can elapse between contact and the development of symptoms.

What are the symptoms?
The main feature of scabies is itch, which is worse at night. Itchy papules are seen on the wrists, hands, nipples, umbilical area and genitals, with little 'burrows' between the fingers. There may be an associated eczema-type rash affecting the skin from the neck downward.

How is it diagnosed?
Generally, the diagnosis is quite evident, with a typical body rash and a history of contact with an affected person. If in doubt, a doctor may open a burrow with the tip of a needle to see if a mite can be extracted.

What are the treatment options?
The affected person, all family/household members and any close contacts should be treated at the same time, whether itching or not. Cream can be obtained from the doctor and it is essential to follow the instructions fully. It is applied prior to going to bed, to the whole body from the neck down. If hands are washed during the night, the cream must be reapplied. The length of application depends on the preparation used. After treatment, all bed linen and clothes should be laundered.

What is the outlook?
The itch may persist for up to a week after treatment, even if it has been successful. However, if new spots are still appearing a week later the treatment will need to be repeated, perhaps using an alternative preparation.

SEBACEOUS CYST
A benign growth under the skin.

Sebaceous cysts form when the release of sebum from the skin is blocked. They are smooth to the touch and range in size, and occur most commonly on the scalp, face, ears and genitals. They only require treatment if they become infected and painful or are excessively large.

SEBORRHOEIC ECZEMA
A type of eczema often only on the scalp, but sometimes on the face, throat, underarm and groin.

What are the causes?
Seborrhoeic eczema is common, with males more often affected than females. The condition is common in adults aged 30–60 and in babies up to the age of 3 months, although affected babies do not necessarily develop the condition in adult life. Originally seborrhoeic eczema was simply thought to be caused by increased sebum production from the sebaceous glands, but it now seems likely that other factors are implicated. *Pityrosporum ovale*, a yeast normally found on the skin, is present in increased numbers, and climate may also play a part as an improvement is often seen in spring and summer. The condition can worsen with stress.

What are the symptoms?
In infants, the most common manifestation is cradle cap, where yellowy-brown, greasy scales adhere to the scalp skin. Scaling may also be evident on the eyebrows, forehead, temple and behind the ears. The nappy area becomes red and scaly, with a clearly defined edge. Infants are generally not distressed by this condition.

In adults, the scaliness may be confined to the scalp, where it is seen as dandruff. However, it may be more widespread, affecting the face, behind the ears, eyelids, chest and back. The groin area and skin beneath the breasts are also commonly affected. Affected skin is generally red, scaly and crusty, and additional infection with yeasts or bacteria is common in both the infant and adult forms.

What are the treatment options?
In infants, the regular use of emollients both as a soap substitute and moisturiser is recommended, including to the nappy area. A mild steroid cream combined with an anti-fungal agent can be used on affected areas if necessary. Frequent shampooing is helpful in lifting the scales on the scalp, and an olive oil scalp massage a couple of hours before shampooing can improve the results.

For adults, frequent use of an anti-yeast shampoo with vigorous massage is helpful, using the lather from the shampoo to wash the body. Steroid creams combined with an anti-infective agent are often used. In widespread or stubborn cases, anti-fungal tablets may be required.

Infants tend to recover by the age of one, but in adults the condition may be chronic, with fluctuations in severity.

SHINGLES (HERPES ZOSTER)
Shingles is caused by the chickenpox virus.

After a bout of chickenpox the virus remains dormant in the nerves and may reactivate at any time to cause shingles, which begins as a burning pain in the skin. This is followed by a crop of blisters along the path of the nerve, which burst and crust. In mild cases, rest and painkillers may be all that is required. Antiviral tablets can be given, but are only effective if started within 48 hours of the rash appearing. Shingles is self-limiting, but ongoing pain after the rash has settled may be a problem. Shingles is contagious: someone who has not had chickenpox may develop it after exposure to shingles.

SQUAMOUS CELL CARCINOMA (SCC)
The second most common type of skin cancer.

What are the causes?
The main cause of SCC is excessive sun exposure. It is more common in outdoor workers and those with outdoor hobbies, especially if fair-skinned. Impairment of the immune system, whether by disease or medication, also increases the likelihood of SCC. The average age of onset is 60–65 years.

What are the symptoms?
SCCs occur in sites that are exposed to the sun (face, ears, the back of the hands). They tend to start as warty nodules or plaques (see actinic keratoses, p. 134) and may thicken and become sore as they grow. The surface is red and crusty and may bleed or ulcerate. They grow steadily and measure from a few millimetres to several centimetres in diameter. Diagnosis is usually suggested by the appearance and confirmed by biopsy or after removal.

What are the treatment options?
The main treatment is surgical removal under anaesthetic. Radiotherapy is also sometimes used. It is important to avoid excess sun, so wearing a hat and long sleeves, and using factor 20 or higher sunscreen when outdoors are necessary.

What is the outlook?
Although spread to other areas of the body is rare, there is an increased chance of spread if the cancer affects the lips or ears. Therefore, anyone affected by SCC needs regular check-ups to ensure the skin remains clear and there is no sign of spread. Most people with SCC are completely cured.

URTICARIA
An itchy red rash, also known as hives or nettle rash.

What are the causes?
Urticaria can be due to a wide range of triggers, including sunlight, cold, pressure, exercise, heat, certain medications and certain foods. It may also indicate an underlying disease. In most cases there is no identifiable cause.

What are the symptoms?
Itchy red plaques, papules or weals with a white centre suddenly arise, often within minutes. Each one may last up to 24 hours then fade without trace. In some cases, swelling of the skin round the eyes and mouth is also seen.

How is it diagnosed?
Biopsy is not generally necessary, as diagnosis can usually be made on the appearance and history. Blood and urine testing plus X-rays may be performed if an underlying illness is suspected.

What are the treatment options?
Any known trigger should be avoided or removed if possible. Aspirin, codeine and any aspirin-based medicines should also be avoided as these are known to worsen urticaria.

Antihistamine tablets should be taken regularly in urticaria of unknown cause. Severe cases may need steroid tablets or referral to a hospital specialist if not settling.

What is the outlook?
Urticaria due to a certain trigger will settle when the cause is removed. Most people will settle over a few months.

VASCULITIS
Inflammation of the blood vessels in the skin or internally.

Vasculitis may be triggered by infection, illness or medication, or be of unknown cause. The lower legs are commonly affected, with painful, purplish spots. If larger blood vessels are affected, the skin ulcerates, and there may be a feeling of malaise if internal blood vessels are affected. A biopsy will confirm skin lesion diagnosis. Blood tests, X-rays and urine analysis may be performed to look for illness. Triggering factors need to be identified and dealt with. In mild cases no treatment may be necessary, however in more severe cases rest is important, and oral steroids may be given.

VITILIGO
A cause of loss of skin pigment.

What are the causes?
Vitiligo affects approximately 1 person in 100, and is caused by a loss of melanocytes in the skin. This is due to an autoimmune disease in which the body attacks its own melanocytes. Other autoimmune diseases may be associated, such as thyroid disease, diabetes and pernicious anaemia. In 30 per cent of cases there is a history of affected family members. All races can be affected.

What are the symptoms?
White areas of skin with a distinct edge are seen, especially around the eyes, mouth, genital region, hands, wrists and knees, and often in a symmetrical pattern. It occurs most commonly in the 20s, although any age groups can be affected. It may be seen first in sites of injury or sunburn. Diagnosis is generally self-evident.

What are the treatment options?
Vitiligo can be a difficult condition to treat successfully and the outlook is unpredictable, as the affected areas may remain static, spread or, rarely, re-pigment. Cosmetics can be used to camouflage the paler areas, and steroid or vitamin D creams may be beneficial. Phototherapy (p. 112) is effective in some cases, although months of treatment may be necessary, and any benefits may be lost when treatment ends. Sunscreen should be used to protect the depigmented area.

WARTS
Warts are caused by the human papilloma virus.

Warts are spread by direct contact with someone who has warts, or via shed patches of skin, for example in swimming pools. It can take a few weeks to several months to develop warts after being in contact with the virus. Verrucas are a form of wart that affects the feet.

What are the symptoms?
The most common type of wart is a firm papule with a rough surface, ranging in size from a few millimetres to over a centimetre in diameter. These are usually found on the hands. Verrucas are often found in groups on the feet.

Flat warts are seen mainly on the face and can be difficult to treat. Warts affecting the anal or genital region should be seen by a doctor.

How is it diagnosed?
Warts are obvious, but in older people they may be mistaken for more serious problems. If in doubt the surface can be scraped to reveal 'black dots' – tiny blood vessels.

What are the treatment options?
Treatment is not essential, as most warts go away eventually if left alone. However, most people prefer to treat warts. Creams are available without prescription. Before application, the wart should be soaked then gently rubbed with a pumice stone or emery board. After drying, the cream is applied to the wart and covered with a plaster. This should be repeated daily. If there is no benefit in 12 weeks, a GP may offer cryotherapy (p. 119).

Warts are rare in babies, common in children and peak at 16–18 years of age, when 20 per cent of young people have at least one.

What is the outlook?
With treatment, 99 per cent of warts will settle eventually. Even with no treatment, it is usual for warts to resolve, although this can take anything from 3 months to 3 years.

XANTHELASMA/XANTHOMA
Raised yellowish papules and plaques on the skin.

These soft yellowish plaques/papules are seen round the eyes (xanthelasma) or other body sites (xanthoma), and are due to deposits of fatty material in the skin. The majority of xanthelasmas are of cosmetic concern only, whereas xanthomas are more likely to be associated with elevated fat and cholesterol levels in the blood. Although diagnosis is clear from their appearance, blood tests should be performed to look for raised cholesterol levels, which may need treatment: the skin lesions usually do not cause problems, but can be treated with trichloracetic acid.

XERODERMA PIGMENTOSUM
The inability of the body to repair sun damage.

This rare genetic disease causes an increased sensitivity to sunlight from infancy, associated with premature ageing of the skin, and the development of skin cancers. Strict sun avoidance is essential and skin cancers must be removed as they occur. Oral treatment may reduce the risk of cancer development. In some cases, lifespan is shortened, but the disease varies greatly in severity.

Index

Acknowledgments

Carroll & Brown Limited would also like to thank:

Picture researcher
Sandra Schneider

Production manager
Karol Davies

Production controller
Nigel Reed

Computer management
Paul Stradling

Indexer
Jill Dormon

3-D anatomy
Mirashade/Matt Gould

Illustrators
Andy Baker, Rajeev Doshi/Regraphica, Kevin Jones Associates, Mikki Rain, John Woodcock

Layout and illustration assistance
Joanna Cameron

Photographers
Jules Selmes, David Yems

Photographic sources
SPL = Science Photo Library

6 *(right)* Getty Images
7 Eye of Science/SPL
8 *(top left)* SPL
10 *(top)* Neil Bromhall/SPL
  (bottom right) Getty Images
11 *(centre)* Sheila Terry/SPL
  (right) Dr P Marazzi/SPL
  (bottom) SPL
12 Gavriel Jecan/Corbis
13 H Raguet/Eurelios/SPL
28 Getty Images
30 Professors P M Motta, K R Porter & P M Andrews/SPL
33 *(left)* Alfred Pasieka/SPL
  (right) Daniel Sambraus/SPL
34 *(top right)* Ken Bank/RetnaUK
34–35 Getty Images
36 Getty Images
36–37 Michael Keller/Corbis
38 *(centre)* Getty Images
  (right) Getty Images
39 Getty Images

40 *(left)* Getty Images
  (top right) Getty Images
  (3rd from top) Getty Images
  (4th from top) Getty Images
  (5th from top) Getty Images
43 Getty Images
44 Getty Images
45 Getty Images
46 *(bottom left)* Getty Images/ Eyewire
47 *(centre, right)* Getty Images
48 Getty Images
49 Getty Images
51 Getty Images
53 Getty Images
55 Getty Images
59 *(top)* Getty Images
60 Getty Images
61 Ellipse Pulsed Light Ltd, 45-47 Cheval Place, London SW7 1EW www.3d.dk
62 Getty Images
70 Getty Images
73 *(top right)* Getty Images/Eyewire
  (bottom right) Getty Images
74 Getty Images
76 Getty Images
77 *(background, top, top right)* Getty Images
  (bottom) Advanced Safety Devices www.safety-devices.com
78 *(top)* Getty Images
  (centre) Peter Scoones/SPL
  (bottom) Getty Images/Eyewire
79 Getty Images
80 Getty Images/Eyewire
81 Getty Images
82 Getty Images
83 *(top right, 3rd from top)* Getty Images
84 *(left, centre right, right)* Getty Images
85 T H Foto-Werbung/SPL
87 Getty Images
92 Getty Images
93 Melle Stripp www.allthingsnails.co.uk
94 Getty Images
100 *(left)* Saturn Stills/SPL
  (centre) Dr Arthur Tucker/SPL
  (right) Eye of Science/SPL
101 David Parker/SPL
104 Dr A Chu
107 *(top)* Dr A Chu
  (bottom) Dr P Marazzi/SPL
108 John Durham/SPL
109 St John's Institute of Dermatology

110 *(top)* Saturn Stills/SPL
  (bottom) SPL
111 David Parker/SPL
112 St John's Institute of Dermatology
113 Jim Selby/SPL
116 Eye of Science/SPL
117 *(top)* Eye of Science/SPL
  (bottom) SPL
118 Getty Images
119 AntoniaReeve/SPL
120 Dr Chris Hale/SPL
121 Dr P Marazzi/SPL
122 Mike Devlin/SPL
123 James Stevenson/SPL
124 *(top)* Dr P Marazzi/SPL
  (bottom) Tony McConnell/SPL
125 Belle Santé UK Ltd www.beauty-guild.co.uk
126 BSIP Laurent H Americain/SPL
127 Wellcome Trust Medical Photographic Library
128 Dr Brian Coghlan
129 Dr Brian Coghlan
130 Dr Arthur Tucker/SPL
131 *(top)* Dr P Marazzi/SPL
  (centre) SimonFraser/NCCT, Freeman Trust, Newcastle-upon-Tyne/SPL
  (bottom) Dr P Marazzi/SPL
132 *(top)* James Stevenson/SPL
  (bottom) Nancy Kedersha/ Immunogen/SPL

Back cover *(right)* Jim Selby/SPL

Contact details
NHS Direct 0845 4647
www.nhsdirect.nhs.uk

Skin Camouflage Service
British Red Cross Association
9 Grosvenor Crescent
London SW1X 7EJ
020 7325 5454

British Association of Aesthetic Plastic Surgeons (BAAPS)
www.baaps.org.uk
(for details of reputable cosmetic surgeons)